繩縛本事

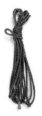

ESSENCE of SHIBARI

Kinbaku and Japanese Rope Bondage

繩縛本事

by Shin Nawakiri

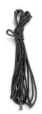

Notice

Essence of Shibari: Kinbaku and Japanese Rope Bondage
by Shin Nawakiri

© 2017 – English Edition – Mystic Productions Press
© 2013 – G Books Taiwan

Original text and rope work by Shin Nawakiri
http://bittersweet.asia/

Photography by Piez Jeng
http://piezphoto.com/

Forward by Nawashi Kanna
http://nawashikanna78.blog136.fc2.com/

Translated and Edited by David Z. and Lee Harrington
http://www.PassionAndSoul.com

English Edition layout and cover by Rob River
www.RobRiver.com

ISBN 978-1-942733-85-0

Ebooks: MOBI – ISBN 978-1-942733-86-7
ePub – ISBN 978-1-942733-87-4
PDF – ISBN 978-1-942733-88-1

Collector's Edition – ISBN 978-1-942733-89-8

Previous/Chinese Language 繩縛本事 978-986-6474-45-3

Foreword

この本の著者と出会ったのは数年前になる。

縛りを覚えたいと言うことで私の元に来て一生懸命縄を覚えていたのを
今でもよく覚えている。

その頃神凪一門と言う一門を設立し、著者にも声をかけ一門入りし、ま
すます縄の技術を身に付けるようになる。

日本の中でも著者の縄の腕前はかなりのものだ。

ここ数年著者には会っていないが、ネットで著者の縛りを見るたびにそ
の頃を懐かしく思うのと同時に、

縄のレベルがあの頃より格段に上がっていてすごく嬉しく思う。

今回緊縛教本を出すということで著者から話を聞いて私自身すごく楽し
みにしている。

この本を読んで皆さんが安全に楽しめる事を願う。

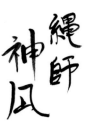

Several years ago I met the author of this book. I still remember the moment when he first came to me to study kinbaku, and his persistent enthusiasm. When Kanna Ichi-mon (the Kanna school of kinbaku) was established, Shin Nawakiri joined us at my invitation. He improved his kinbaku skills, and his skill level was very good even compared to those in Japan.

Although I have not reunited with the author in the past few years, when I see his kinbaku work on the internet, I reminisce over those past days of us together, and feel very happy that his kinbaku level has further advanced to a higher level.

Now, as I hear about his upcoming publication of this book, I am also filled with anticipation, and very much hope that all those who will read this book will learn kinbaku in a safe and joyful way.

Nawashi Kanna

Editor and Translator's Notes

It has been an honor to get a chance to bring Shin Nawakiri's book, *Essence of Shibari: Kinbaku and Japanese Rope Bondage*, to an English-speaking audience. Ever since I saw the book, I knew it was something special, and set upon an almost two year quest into making it happen.

This book offered unique challenges in that it was written in Chinese, by an author from Taiwan, about a topic (and teachings) originating from Japan. The author cited works from teachers that speak English, Italian, and Spanish – providing additional hoops for confirming correct translation of their quotes. We chose to list all of the above languages in English for the book: Japanese-language concepts that were listed in rōmaji (roman letters) with translations listed as [translation] after them; and Chinese-language specific terms listed as the English translation followed by the original Chinese characters.

Another choice we debated were the words 'kinbaku' and 'shibari'. In Chinese, these words get used interchangeably, as was the case in classical magazines such as Kitan Club from the 1950s. In current English vernacular, shibari often gets used to refer to Westernized Japanese aesthetic ropework, while kinbaku is used for Japanese work done in Japan. However, both terms are used in Japan at this time. We have chosen to use both terms interchangeably in the early parts of this book, shifting later in the book to kinbaku to reference the style and tool, and shibari to reference specific ties.

One of the reasons that Nawakiri's book was specifically of interest to us at Mystic Productions Press was that it features both male and female bodies being bound. That is not the case in the work of all authors, who tend to feature a specific aesthetic of the female body. When a he or she is referenced in this book, it is referring to the gender of the person in the images, not a tie being limited to a specific gender. Though the book features Taiwanese models, these ties can all be modified for diverse bodies, and Nawakiri says that no reader needs to feel excluded from the ties, even if not all body types are directly shown.

The original text features a number of Taiwanese-specific references. Some have been kept for interest of the reader, while others have been modified – with author permission – to open the topics to a Western audience. Some safety ties have also been expanded for awareness that may have been previously understood by his original audience.

In doing all of this play, please remember that one of the basic tenets of shibari is that it requires active informed consent between adults. This includes awareness of personal safety and discussing the needs, wants, and desires of all parties. It is wonderful to have a rich text like this one to share, but understand that all ideas, techniques, and notes on safety and technique are from but one perspective, and there are others out there. We encourage readers do their own research and look into other works, as well.

We hope that you will enjoy this work as much as we do, and dive into the beautiful world of kinbaku with Shin Nawakiri as your guide.

Yours in rope and joy,

David Z. and
Lee Harrington

TABLE OF CONTETS

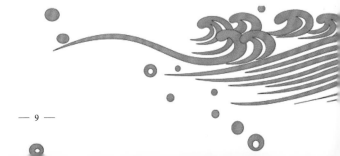

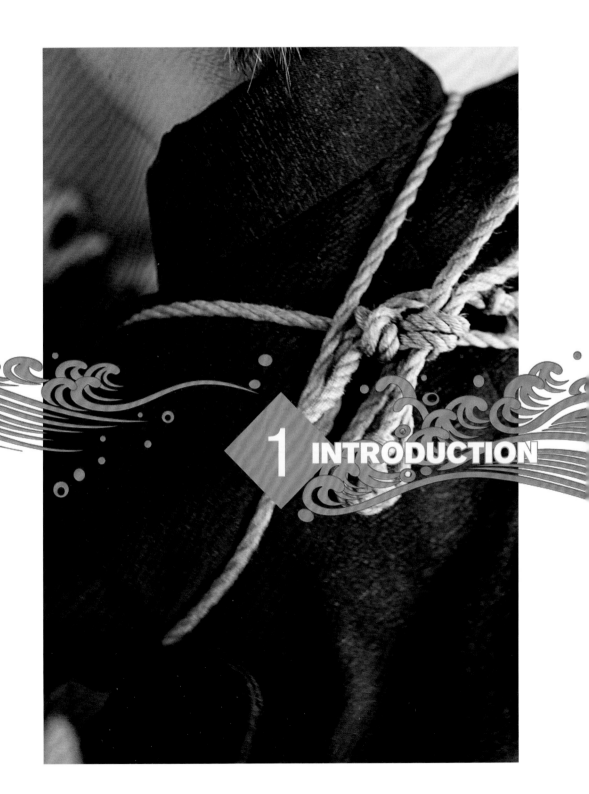

1 INTRODUCTION

Some people see kinbaku as a beautiful and cruel expression of sexual desire, while others see it as a refined performance art. Whichever view you may hold, kinbaku – also known as shibari – has become a symbol of Japanese SM.

Since the Second World War, BDSM communities in the West have explored and defined concepts such as Dominant, submissive, Top, bottom, and other related terminology. By doing so, they have established a foundation for the long-term development of a BDSM subculture. However, in Japan, there seems to be a lack of this kind of social movement. Fans of SM explore this aspect of their sexuality through videos and books, as well as through watching bakushi [rope bondage masters, teachers, or artists] talk about their profession, their experiences in the SM lifestyle, and their understanding of roles of SM practitioners. Accordingly, bakushi have played a very influential part in the forming of Japanese SM subculture.

Kinbaku has also become popular among BDSM circles in the West since the turn of the century. Aficionados from all over the world have formed interest and practice groups, and some have made pilgrimages to Japan to study this art. Well-known bakushi have become international celebrities. Meanwhile, BDSM circles in the West have continued their longstanding tradition of sharing and publicizing knowledge. The flourishing community-based kink culture has established an efficient network to share knowledge on shibari.

As a result, in the past decade, the level of kinbaku accomplishment in the West has advanced rapidly. I believe that the top players in the West have remarkably attained the same level of quality as those well-known bakushi in Japan, and a number of upcoming aficionados in the West are equally remarkable. With a high level in both quality and quantity, Western kinbaku circles already have the ability to rely on themselves to explore, comprehend, and develop new skills of kinbaku.

Taiwan and other Chinese-speaking regions benefit from a proximity to Japan, and subsequentially have been in contact with kinbaku earlier than the West. However, whereas the West has advanced greatly thus far, the Chinese-speaking regions have been relatively slow to pick up kinbaku. Perhaps this is because the BDSM circles in the Chinese-speaking regions are not as enthusiastic as their counterparts in Japan and the West. In addition, there is a lack of teaching materials written in Chinese. Although there are many people who are interested in kinbaku and hope to learn, it has been difficult for them to find suitable channels and resources.

The original Chinese-language title of this book was 繩縛本事, which can be roughly translated as Kinbaku Skills. The term "skills" conveys a sense of abilities and techniques. However, the Chinese character for "skills" also means basics, which conveys a sense of being at the foundation or origin of things. Thus, for this translation we have chosen the name Essence of Shibari: Kinbaku and Japanese Rope Bondage – because at the end of the day it is this essence that is being conveyed.

I hope this book may guide its readers to practice the basics of kinbaku, help newcomers to get started, and enrich the experience of established enthusiasts. Ever since shibari has become popular, much of its exploration has been ongoing without an end in sight. Old knowledge is being challenged, new theories are being discussed, and novel techniques are being developed. In this book I will strive to introduce the new knowledge and skills that I have learned, along with my personal understanding of kinbaku. Ideally it will be of some help to the readers that want to study kinbaku, encouraging more people to start to practice and play.

As more fellow kinksters learn from each other, their skills will surely improve faster. As more of these kinksters play with rope at various venues, the wider public may see what they do and become interested. Even if those interested observers do not start playing with rope themselves, they may still develop a capacity to appreciate and enjoy rope scenes. In this way, our kinbaku circles will only get bigger, leading to more possibilities for good things to happen in the future.

Shin Nawakiri

1.1 What Can This Book Teach You?

When I started studying kinbaku in 2003, during a class, Nawashi Kanna asked students to discuss why they wanted to study kinbaku. Is it for playing with their partners? Or is it for use during SM domination sessions? Is it for taking beautiful photographs? Or is it for performance on stage?

For different purposes, the direction of study and method of techniques will be different. Playful bondage between partners does not require knowledge of complicated techniques – what is needed is a sense of closeness between each other. In SM domination sessions, suffering created within a range of control by rope is called "semenawa," and it requires more knowledge concerning safety. Command of time and tempo is also key. For creating photographic images, it is necessary to pay attention to details, but not necessary to bring theatric showmanship to the bondage process.

On-stage performance requires both speed and force; also, the nawashi must learn how to avoid blocking the audience's line of sight by stepping away from the model. The audience purchased tickets to see a show, desiring to see something more than what bedroom-time can offer. Therefore, on-stage performance often shows the extremes, challenging the limit of both the nawashi and the model. Nawashi can only strive for, as much as they can, a balance between showing a spectacle and taking into account the comfort of the model.

I hope this book can satisfy the different needs of its various readers. Those that hope to apply a little bondage to make sex and domination more fun, or those that hope to accomplish beautiful static shibari, will be able to learn the necessary techniques and safety knowledge. For those that want to study difficult on-stage kinbaku performance skills or semenawa, this book also offers some of those related techniques that will serve as a foundation for further study. For those that are purely curious about kinbaku and are not thinking about actually doing the bondage, this book will teach you how to enjoy and appreciate the art of kinbaku.

Many people in the BDSM community have this misconception that they should aim to tie up someone so tightly that it will be impossible to get out of the tie. They think, to truly immobilize the person being tied, not only should the tie be tight, it should also make that person uncomfortable. Hojojutsu, a martial art that originated ancient Japan, uses a single thin rope to bite into the body to cause pain during struggle, wrap around the arms to numb the nerves, and circle around the neck to impair breathing. As a result, the prisoner would feel pain or dizziness as soon as he moves, which would prevent escape. Every such principle of hojojutsu is exactly opposite to the basic rules of modern shibari. Like all SM practices, shibari also requires informed consent between partners. Therefore, modern SM bondage regards the ability to create a sense of restraint without causing too much discomfort of the bottom or bound partner as a basic skill. Doing so makes it possible to prolong play time.

Nawashi Stefano Laforgia has come up with a clever metaphor: "Teaching kinbaku is like teaching cooking." After teaching the basic skills, the teacher can only tell you how some of the things you do might be wrong. For example, adding salt to coffee is probably not a good idea. But how should one make things better? Everyone has his own style in cooking, so to judge whether a dish is good or not, the criteria is not whether or not the cook has accurately followed a recipe. Only those who have tasted your cooking are qualified to judge.

You and your partner must find the kinbaku dishes that work for both of you. Chapter 2 will briefly introduce the basic knowledge of rope, its recognition and methods of treatment. After that, we will introduce in Chapter 3 a saying that falls on one end of the spectrum of kinbaku practice: "You may practice kinbaku without using any knots, but you cannot practice kinbaku without putting in your emotion." This is the soul and spirit of kinbaku.

Chapter 4 continues to introduce basic skills that are often used in kinbaku. Individually, these knots may look plain and simple, but when used in combination they can produce all sorts of variations. At the end of this chapter we will do a comprehensive exercise to let the reader apply these basic skills to produce some unexpected decorative patterns of macramé.

Before advancing to higher levels of ties, in Chapter 5 we will call reader's attention to those precautions that kinbaku participants should know. These include technical items – simple anatomical knowledge and selection of body parts to apply the rope, as well as psychological aspects – how to choose your kinbaku partner, knowing thyself, and things that need to be communicated to each other. This chapter is important to read for both those tying and those being bound.

From Chapter 6 onward we will introduce common kinbaku ties one by one. Some ties are suitable to be used in SM play and domination, whereas others are more difficult kinbaku foundation ties. We allocate the introduction of the first major obstacle to studying modern Japanese kinbaku – takate kote, also known as TK – in Chapter 7 alone. If you only do kinbaku for fun, or only perform the ties on the ground, then you may get away with only the basic concept for your sessions. Full suspension demands a relatively high level of requirement for precision and detail. This chapter is presented according to the standards of full suspension. Chapter 8 will introduce practical applications of kinbaku in our everyday environment by utilizing furniture and tools, as well as a brief presentation of semenawa.

Full suspension that lifts a person off the floor is often seen in performances, as well as being possibly used in semenawa. These advanced techniques involve factors such as buildup of sophisticated psychological milieu, such as pre-suspension preparation by Top and bottom, quick response to developments during suspension, and aftercare. It would easily take a dedicated book to discuss this topic alone. After much reflection, I have decided not to teach full suspension in this book, hoping to fully cover this topic in the future. Individuals who want to learn these skills are encouraged to seek out teachers who have extensive knowledge in the field. However, every chapter of this book – including safety precautions and details of TK techniques – is presented according to the standard applicable to full suspension. On one hand, this allows the students of kinbaku skills to do so in a more rigorous way; on the other hand, this also allows those being tied to understand the necessary standard in order to protect their own safety.

While studying these skills, some students may inevitably lose their perspective, being distracted by what they are learning. Many nawashi emphasize the principle that "techniques are secondary, while all variations depend on the mother wit." This may sound easy, but to me it is a wisdom only realized after my learning has gone full circle.

The harder the kinbaku technique, the more reflective it is of the relationship between the tying partners. Often a bottleneck is confronted when a knot cannot be completed, when the tightness of rope is misjudged, or when the Top gets a little bit slow, thereby causing pain to the bottom. At such a moment, the various past displeasures between the two, the suppressed emotions, and the dust-laden memories begin to surface. By taking a moment to let your eyes connect, that expression lets your partner know and accept the other's feelings, such that the nawashi feels the pain suffered by the model and is filled with gratitude, while the model in turn feels that all the pain is worth it. Thus the two appreciate what they are striving to achieve. Working together in a seamless way to arrive at the moment when the two hearts connect – this is more precious than anything.

All this is not that hard to understand; a couple that practices intensely as dance partners will be able to share the same experience. The only difference is that in kinbaku, the bakushi and the model are involving themselves in a more extreme challenge. Learning shibari is a journey where both people grow together. Books, the internet, and kinbaku teachers can only set you upon your own path of learning. The one that will teach you the most is still your partner. I hope that you, the kinbaku practitioners will treasure your partners, and always hold gratitude to them; for they are spending their time to teach us with their bodies.

Although not all readers will dig into kinbaku topics of the most difficult levels, I hope that your journey of growth is one that is worth your effort.

1.2 History of Kinbaku

Connecting restraint, sadomasochism, and sexual desire is a basic instinct. The way to put such desire to practice naturally draws inspiration from each person's cultural environment.

Due to historical factors, objects such as handcuffs, shackles, metal restraints, leather, and latex clothing, have become representative elements of BDSM in the West. In Japan, rope and tying are originally part of daily lives. For example, shime nawa [the rope used to cordon off consecrated areas or as a talisman against evil] hangs inside Shinto shrines; while kimonos don't have buttons, and instead have several inner and outer layers that are all tied with belts. Thus, in Japan, prisoners were naturally tied with ropes.

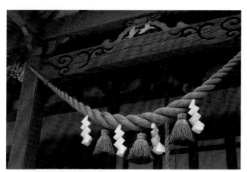

Shime Nawa. Aichi Prefecture Okazaki City Yamanaka Hachiman Shrine. Photo by Paul Davidson.

According to historical research, there is also this following theory: In ancient time, Japan lacked iron, so Doushin [peace officers] did not have handcuffs like their Western or Chinese counterparts. In the Edo period from 1603 to 1868, Japan developed more than 150 schools of hojojutsu. People from different social stations were tied using different methods. Various regions have their own ways of tying in order to distinguish their jurisdictions. The many techniques and styles of hojojutsu have profoundly influenced modern Japanese kinbaku.

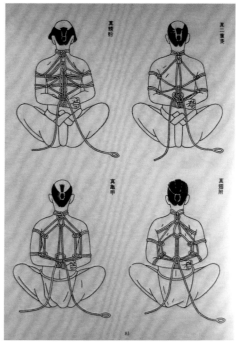

Hojojutsu, Ittatsu Ryu School, "Shin Nijuu Hishi" [true double diamond] and "Shin Tonbo" [real dragonfly] ties. Zukai Hojoujutsu by Fujita Seiko.

On the other hand, human nature has an innate curiosity towards spectacles of cruelty and torture. Many theatrical programs of traditional kabuki, including the famous classical operas of "Yuki-me" [Snow Maiden] and "Kinkaku-ji" [Temple of the Golden Pavilion, a Zen Buddhist temple in Kyoto], all contain plots of Seme-ba that depict the leading roles suffering from beating and torture. From the mid-Meiji Period, a type of drama called "Soushi Shibai" [Hero's Drama] was developed. Originally, it was meant to depict heroes revolting against oppression from the regime, and to advocate freedom and civil rights. Later, it took on a political stance that increasingly leaned towards establishing the nation and state, while its dramatic plot adopted more and more scenes of torture. Politics, sex, and violence fed off each other; a phenomenon that is not that uncommon among many nations' plebian culture.

After the First Sino-Japanese War, in June of 1896, the Hongo Haruki-za Theater in Tokyo put on stage a drama called "Nisshin Senso – Yon-chi no Kataki-tan" [First Sino-Japanese War – Tale of the Enemy's Night Attack]. It depicted several Japanese nurses being tortured and humiliated by Chinese soldiers in Manchuria – but given their noble virtue – forgave their tormentors. This piece of drama took advantage of the protective umbrella of nationalism, and used it as a pretext to showcase sexual cruelty. It profoundly touched a fourteen-year-old young man among the audience. Many years later, he would, under the *nom de guerre* of Ito Seiu, become a kinbaku painter, photographer, and research investigator. He published the first

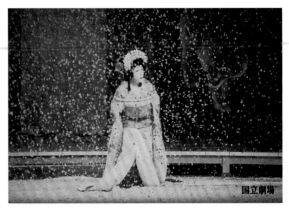

"Gion Sairei Shinkou Ki" [Tale of the Gion Festival] Snow Maiden as acted by Nakamura Jakuemon IV. November, 1997. National Theater.

photo-book of kinbaku in Japan named "Seme no Kenkyu" [Study of Torture] in 1928, and organized theater shows. Eventually, he became recognized as the father of modern Japanese kinbaku.

It is worth noticing that "Seme no Kenkyu" is a study of torture. The terms "sadism" and "masochism" only became widely used in Japan in the 1950s. The term BDSM – acronym for bondage, discipline, sadism and masochism – was only invented in the West in the 1980s. It stands to reason that, before these terms became widely known there, the Japanese interpretation of BDSM was based on torture. This is "beauty in suffering" that is deep-rooted in Japanese style esthetics, depicting a release of emotion in a poignant and cruel context. It is a tradition that is different from the BDSM culture in the West. Kinbaku is one of the various torture methods. Tying up someone not only prevents escape, but can also be used for humiliation and torment. Suspending, pulling, or contorting the body and muscles can all cause pain and suffering. Nowadays, there are those that take the words too literally, and classify kinbaku under bondage and discipline of BDSM. In fact, the two practices have different threads of thought, and are difficult to discuss under the same framework.

The postwar '50s and '60s is the heyday of the magazine Kitan Club [Club of Strange Tales]. This magazine often used sex, torture, abuse, and exotic customs as its main themes, with occasional detective stories or even science fiction. It subtly pointed to some alternative styles of taste and preference, but is difficult to classify and generalize according to today's rigid approach. From today's point of view, this magazine can be regarded as a precious historical representative of the formative period of Japanese SM culture. In addition, Kitan Club also acted as a promoter of kinbaku culture. Suma Toshiyuki, who worked as a writer, illustrator, and photographer, along with people such as Tsujimura Takashi

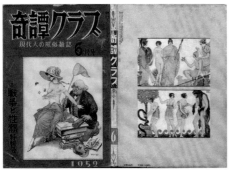

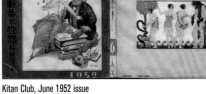

Kitan Club, June 1952 issue

[the two people collectively used more than ten pseudonyms in order to create an impression of many authors], first researched kinbaku for the purpose of illustration. With the improvement of printing technology, their magazines also began to publish works of photography. It is believed that the term "nawashi" was first used in the '50s by Tsujimura Takashi in his magazines. In 1962, Dan Oniroku's novel "Hana to Ebi" [Flower and Snake] began its serial publication in Kitan Club.

In 1965, Osada Eikichi amazed the world with a single brilliant feat: an SM experimental drama, which is now widely acknowledged as the progenitor of kinbaku stage performance. In his heyday, his performance could command a high price of ten thousand yen per ticket. From the late '60s to early '70s, with the popularization of "Pink Cinema" type movies, people like Konuma Takashi also began to assume the role of kinbaku directors in movie productions. In 1974, facing impending bankruptcy, Nikkatsu film company decided to make "Flower and Snake" as one last throw of the dice and achieved unexpected popularity. Afterwards, the movie's kinbaku director Urado Hiroshi collaborated with Nikkatsu on a total of 46 movies. In order to safely adapt kinbaku to its newly found applications

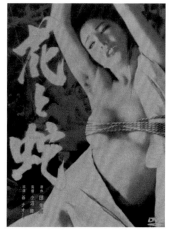

Flower and Snake (1974), distributed by Nikkatsu. Written by Dan Oniroku, directed by Konuma Masaru; Kinbaku direction by Urado Hiroshi

in photography, stage performance and movies without harming the models, they experimented with all kinds of new kinbaku techniques that captured the verve and charm of kabuki and hojojutsu, while taking into account safety issues. From several decades of records starting from Kitan Club, we can see the modern kinbaku techniques gradually taking shape during this period.

With the advent of VHS tapes in the '80s, adult videos gradually replaced adult films. Nawashi such as Nureki Chimuo, Shima Shikou, Akechi Denki, and Arisue Go not only assisted in the kinbaku production of adult movies, but also became a new generation of celebrities. In addition to granting appearances and demonstrating kinbaku techniques, these community celebrities also had opportunities to get vocal on issues. They appeared in movies, speaking with fervor and assurance, talking about what rope means to them, their emotional connections with their models, and the true meaning of SM as they see it. These words by the nawashi have come to nourish generations of Japanese SM enthusiasts, and have exerted an important force to influence and shape the SM culture in Japan.

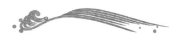

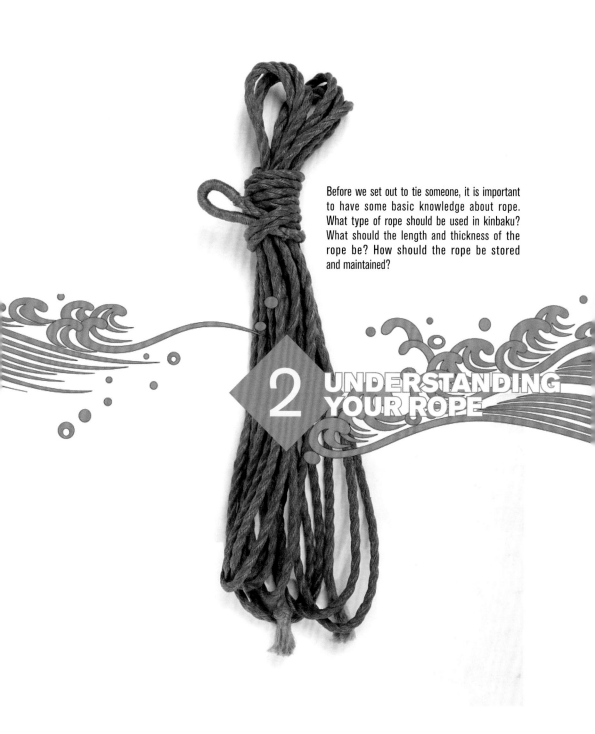

Before we set out to tie someone, it is important to have some basic knowledge about rope. What type of rope should be used in kinbaku? What should the length and thickness of the rope be? How should the rope be stored and maintained?

2 UNDERSTANDING YOUR ROPE

2.1 Materials and Specifications

The Style of Rope

The use of hemp rope is one of the distinguishing features of modern Japanese kinbaku. Hemp rope has a rough texture, which enables the creation of friction tightened knots in kinbaku application. It also lacks elasticity, which lets the nawashi rely on the feeling of his hands to control the level of tightness of the wraps, and also reduces deforming the rope when under pressure. The many techniques of Japanese kinbaku have all been developed based on the hemp rope.

However, "hemp rope" is used as a collective term – ropes made of fibers from several different genus of plants all look like hemp rope to an average person, and might fall under this description. Within the kinbaku community in Japan, jute is often used. In Europe and America, rope made from marijuana hemp fiber is relatively easy to obtain. In recent years, people have tried linen rope, which has a delicate feel to it. Manila and sisal rope can be bought from hardware stores, but their textures are tough and are difficult to soften, and thus are not suitable for use in kinbaku.

Cotton rope has a texture that is softer than hemp, and is elastic. Its advantage is its relatively comfortable feel to the skin as compared with hemp rope. Its drawback is its tendency to stretch under tension. For one thing, it is quite difficult to control the level of tightness. For another, when under powerful tension, its knots will tighten and become difficult to undo. Cotton rope does not easily absorb lubricating oil, and when it is dry, the rope is abrasive to the tier's fingers. Still, many individuals prefer cotton rope for its ease of use.

Nylon rope has been widely used for bondage in Europe and America. The surface of nylon rope has a smoother texture than natural fiber ropes, so the techniques to create knots and to affix the ropes to one another are different from those used with hemp rope. Compared with natural fiber, one of the advantages of nylon rope is that it does not shrink in water. Therefore, for photography or domination sessions in bathrooms or at the beach, the rope can still be safely used even after being soaked in water.

The so-called "boy scout rope" available in Taiwan is probably made from either nylon, or polyester, or perhaps cotton. Its toughness, elasticity, length, and thickness are not consistent. You need to ascertain its specifications before purchase.

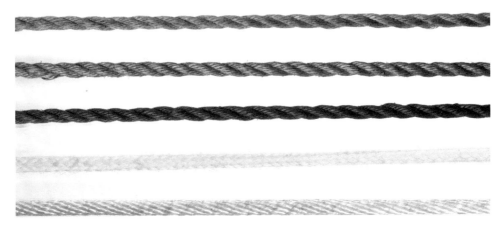

From top to bottom: natural color jute rope, hemp rope dyed azure and red, cotton rope, and nylon rope.

Length and Amount

Modern Japanese kinbaku uses hemp rope with a length of 7.5 to 8 meters (24-26 feet), and a diameter of 6 mm (1/4 inch). Japanese Bakushi usually prepare several ropes of the same specification. Ropes that have different lengths and thickness are used on special occasions as supplements. Westerners have larger bodies, so some people have experimented with using 8 mm (1/3 inch) hemp rope as their primary rope.

Creative practices of kinbaku can have many variations without using many ropes. For example, a widely popular "One Rope" technique uses only one piece of rope to bring into play the essence of kinbaku. The relatively complicated upper body ties may use up to three pieces of ropes. In general, five pieces of rope should be sufficient to tie both upper and lower bodies. My own habit is to use a larger set comprised of ten pieces of 6 mm wide, 8 meter long, ropes. This should be enough to deal with most on-stage performances.

Where to Buy

Before buying anything referred to as "hemp rope," you should first find out about its material. It is hard to obtain jute or hemp from regular hardware stores. I suggest you purchase hemp rope from specialty rope stores [that cater to the general public instead of SM clientele], and process the ropes yourselves with the methods taught in this book. Ropes sold at sex toy shops are several times more expensive, and their qualities are often not consistent, which may require further processing in order to be usable. There are stores in Japan that specialize in the sale of processed kinbaku ropes, with their even more exorbitant prices. However, if you have tried using those complicated procedures to process ropes, you may agree that it is reasonable to sell well-processed ropes at high prices. There are many online stores now, especially in the West, that sell processed ropes with a variety of prices and varying quality.

For those readers who do not have the means to acquire hemp rope, or who are not in a position to process hemp rope, rope of other materials but with the same thickness and length may be a temporary substitute. To those who are being tied, soft-feeling cotton rope may be more comfortable. This book will also discuss using the relatively smooth nylon rope to make a single column tie and to connect to another piece of rope.

Processing

Regardless of which channel has been used to purchase the hemp rope, the rope may still be too rough and stiff, and needs to go through several processing steps that include boiling, straightening, singeing, and oiling in order to be made suitable for kinbaku. Bakushi usually process ropes themselves in Japan, while many in the West are choosing to support rope bondage vendors. We will introduce in details the treatment and maintenance of ropes in Section 2.4. Processing hemp rope is a time-consuming art that requires a lot of effort, but after being properly processed, the rope goes up in value considerably.

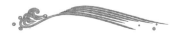

2.2 Language Specification

Rope Bottom: The terms "m-male," "m-female," or "slave" are often used to call the partner who is being tied. In performance circles, the terms "rope model" or "kinbaku model" are used. Since both these terms are not completely suitable in kinbaku practices – the person being tied is not necessarily a masochist or slave, or a rope model performing on stage – this book uses the term "Rope Bottom."

Rope Top: When I first began to study kinbaku, the term "nawashi" was an honorific title for an esteemed Top in the kinbaku circle, but it cannot be used to refer to oneself. This book uses the term "rope Top" for the person who does the tying.

Rope head, rope tail: Rope is often folded in half and then used. This enlarges the area where the rope contacts the body, thereby increasing comfort. Therefore, as tying begins, the usable working length of the rope is approximately 3.7 to 4 meters (12-13 feet). After being folded in half, the section originally at the center of the rope is called the "rope head" or "bight," and the two original ends of the rope now becomes the "rope tail." Usually the tie begins by using the rope head, whereas the two pieces of rope forming the rope tail will each have a knot. After the rope is used up, this knotted rope tail may be used to connect to the rope head of the next rope.

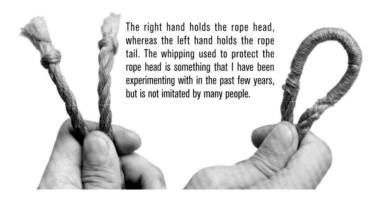

The right hand holds the rope head, whereas the left hand holds the rope tail. The whipping used to protect the rope head is something that I have been experimenting with in the past few years, but is not imitated by many people.

Working end, rope head end: This book follows the custom of regular rope art and knot textbooks, and uses the term "working end" or "free end" to call the end of the rope that is being manipulated and is moving. Only under rare circumstances (often at the beginning of the tying) are both the rope head and the rope tail ends simultaneously manipulated. At such a time, we will use the term "rope head end" and "rope tail end." This book uses the terms "end" and "section" interchangeably, with the former term emphasizing a point, and the latter term emphasizing a rope segment.

Dominant hand, non-dominant hand: When explaining some detailed techniques, we will try to accommodate both right-handed and left-handed readers. We will refer to the right hand of a right-handed person as "dominant hand," and the other hand as "non-dominant hand."

2.3 Storage of Rope

The best way to store rope is to fold it and hang it in a cool, well-ventilated place, while keeping the rope straight. If living conditions do not allow the rope to be hung, then we have to bundle it to be stored. During travel and before performances, ropes should also be bundled to be later undone one by one. Storing rope often starts with the rope tail, so that when undoing the rope, the rope head may be immediately located. The following introduces a rope storage method.

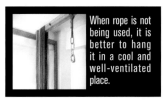
When rope is not being used, it is better to hang it in a cool and well-ventilated place.

1

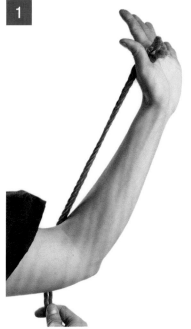

2

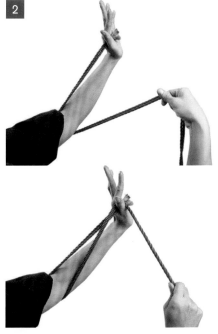

1 Use the Tiger Mouth [the web between thumb and index finger] of the non-dominant hand to hold the rope tail, such that the rope tail is situated at the palm

2 Hook the rope around the elbow of the non-dominant hand, from the outside to the inside, and return the rope to the inner forearm; then hook the rope around the thumb from outside to the inside.

3

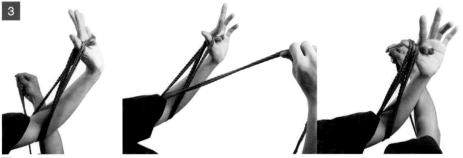

3 Hook the rope around the elbow of the non-dominant hand, this time from the inside to the outside, and return the rope to the outer forearm; then hook the rope around the thumb, this time from the inside to the outside.

4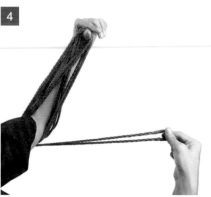

5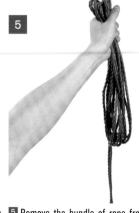

4 Repeat steps 3 and 4, until the length of the rope head end is approximate the length between the Tiger Mouth and the elbow.

5 Remove the bundle of rope from the elbow, and hold the bundle with the non-dominant hand.

6

7

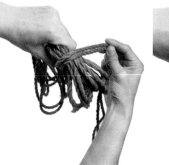 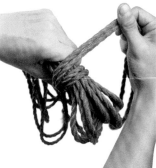 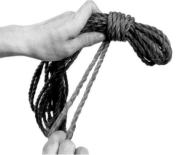

6 Using the dominant hand, wrap the rope head end around the rope bundle once. When returning to the starting position of the wrap, cross over to squeeze the root of the starting position.

7 Continue wrapping in one direction, until the rope head end has about 20 cm (7.5 inches) left.

8

9

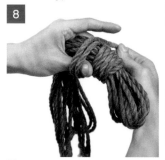 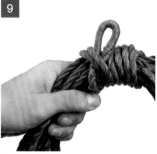

8 Wrap one last time, over the thumb of the non-dominant hand.

9 Pull out the thumb, thereby forming a small opening under the last wrap. Stuff the rope head end through this small opening, and pull tight.

When using the rope, pull out the rope head, and the rope will become unbundled.

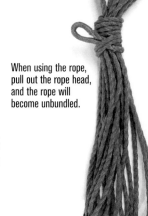

2.4 Treatment and Maintenance of Rope

(1) If the raw rope is purchased as a ball of rope, it is customarily cut into 7.5 to 8 meters (24-26 feet) sections. Most people will tie an overhand knot at each rope tail to prevent its strands from spreading apart, and also to make it easier to connect ropes. The advantage of the overhand knot is its simplicity; the shortcoming is its tendency to come undone (but it is also easy to undo the knot and start over), as well as the relative large knot it forms, which is easy to get stuck. There are also people that use smaller knots, or finish the rope tail without using any knot. Both situations have their own rope connecting methods, which can be found in detail in Chapter 4.5.

There are several ways to finish the end of a rope. From left to right are, overhand knot, wall knot with sailmaker's whipping, wall knot fixed with glue, thistle knot, and sailmaker's whipping without knot (which requires rope connection methods as laid out in Section 4.5.2 or 4.5.3).

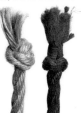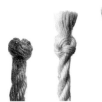

(2) After purchase, the raw rope should be boiled once to soften it. Prepare a large pot, wait for the water to boil, and then fold the raw rope in half several times to put it in. The rope should be submerged in water as much as possible. There are many opinions on how long the rope should be boiled, from 20 minutes to overnight simmering. I often boil the rope for 40 minutes.

Boiling can soften the rope, but also affects the strength of the rope, and shorten its lifespan. I suggest boiling the rope only once.

(3) Place the boiled rope into a washing machine to spin off the water. My suggestion is to place the rope in a lingerie bag to prevent damage to the rope.

(4) Hang the rope in a cool and well-ventilated place to air-dry. It is usually necessary to dry for two days.

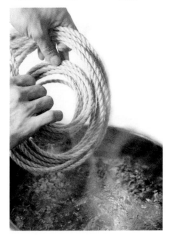

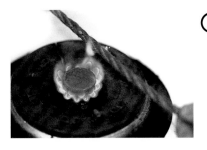

(5) After air-drying, use a low flame to singe off the excess fluff of the rope. It is acceptable to use a candle flame, portable gas stove, or kitchen gas burner. When flaming off the fluff, hold a small section of rope, and rapidly move it back and forth over the flame. Using caution is important with any fire. A decrease of the size of the flame is a sign that most of the fluff has been flamed off, so you can move onto the next section. Be careful not to char the rope.

A meticulous approach to flame off the fluff is to unwind the three strands of each small section of rope with both hands, so that the fluff in the center of the rope can also be flamed off. Others use a relatively rougher approach and hang up the rope, using a large flame or torch to singe off fluff. This is not recommended for indoor spaces, as it can be dangerous. Using a meticulous approach is encouraged, remembering that if the rope produces fluff again, you can repeat less meticulously.

⑥ The next step is to oil and wax the rope. This not only protects the rope bottom, but also protects the rope Top's fingers.

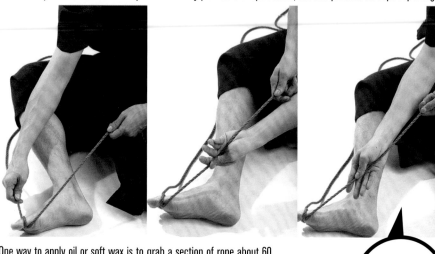

One way to apply oil or soft wax is to grab a section of rope about 60 cm to one meter (2-3 feet) long, use your toe to grip one end of the rope, spread the oil or wax on your palms, and use both hands in turn to wipe it onto the rope. Then move onto the next section. Choices for use include horse oil, baby oil, hemp oil, mink oil, tsubaki oil, coconut oil, jojoba oil, or beeswax. It is not necessary to over-lubricate the rope. After several uses, the rope needs to be oiled and waxed again.

Unprocessed rope (bottom of the image) and jute rope that has been flamed and oiled or waxed (top of the image).

Several commonly found oils and waxes:

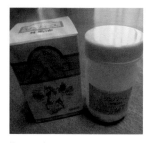

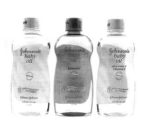

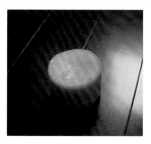

Horse oil: made with animal fat and sold in drug stores. Originally a personal care product to protect hands against dry climate, it is now regarded as the best product for rope lubrication. However, it is quite costly.

Baby oil: a relatively inexpensive choice. Some people mix baby oil with horse oil.

Beeswax: dryer than oil, with very good lubricating effect. Some people mix in oil to make the wax more pliable.

⑦ Before kinbaku, in order to maintain cleanliness, it is advisable to grip the rope with a clean wet cloth, and wipe the rope once.

⑧ In the middle of kinbaku, before pulling on the rope with force, use fingers to grip onto the whole rope in order to prevent pulling apart the three strands of the rope. If the rope is pulled apart, then undo the knot at the rope tail, and rewind the three strands to form the rope again.

(9) In kinbaku the rope is often wiggled back and forth, which can deform the three strands. Each time your play is finished, use one hand to grasp onto the rope, and use the other hand to pull on the rope. Follow the rope's helix pattern to pull the rope straight.

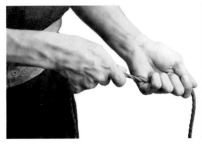 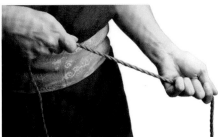

(10) After a period of use, the rope will produce fluff again, so you may need to once again flame off the fluff and apply oil or wax. Also, the rope may be stained with dust, sweat, body fluid, and other things. Cleaning the rope is necessary after some use. Machine washing will easily damage the rope, so it can only be used to spin off water from the rope. Currently the best method seems to be hand-washing the rope first, then spinning off water with a washing machine, followed by air drying.

(11) The rope's most vulnerable place for wear and tear is the rope head. When cracks appear in the rope head, the rope can no longer be used to bear weight. In addition, the body of the rope can sustain wear and tear under tension, and becomes thinner and thinner. When it is thinned too far, it can no longer be used to tie someone, and should be replaced with another rope.

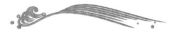

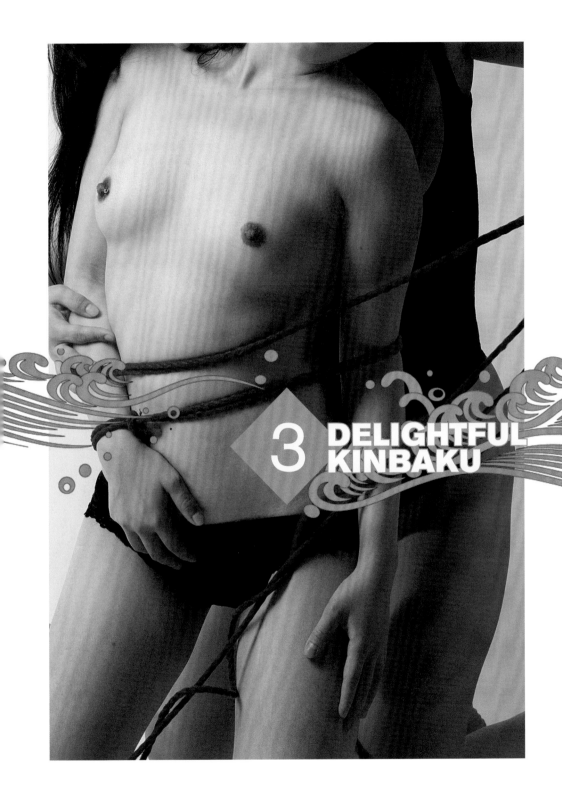

3 DELIGHTFUL KINBAKU

There are only a few techniques used in kinbaku, but these basic ties each require memorizing the way the rope moves. In addition, a student will need to learn how to apply force when tying, and become comfortable with the rope in their hand. Kinbaku students will inevitably get caught up in the techniques and become lost. Paying too much attention to the techniques leads to neglecting your partner – effectively "seeing the rope while missing the person" – creating a bottleneck to learning. It then becomes necessary to intentionally forget, to discard what you have learned, in order to reclaim your original intention when you first began learning kinbaku.

Therefore, I intend to use this chapter as the first lesson of our kinbaku study: kinbaku should be an expression of sexual desire and love; it is a way for two people to communicate with each other, and to mutually enjoy the experience. Playing with rope may be done with almost no techniques or skills, but it cannot be done without this spirit.

The concept of this chapter is inspired by the "One Rope" technique. This style of thinking has been suggested by nawashi Wykd Dave and others. I learned this technique in classes by Hedwig Ve. One Rope technique advocates discarding complex techniques, and using only one rope without making knots or connecting rope. With the hope to minimize the requirement for techniques, it refocuses attention from the rope back to the partner.

The content of this chapter is suitable for those partners that have mutually established emotional basis and closeness, while not rejecting bodily contact.

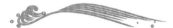

Select a quiet, comfortable, and relaxing location. You can play music that both of you like. Establish a serene environment. Being able to hear each other's breathing and the sound of the rope is ideal.

Unbundle a rope, and place it within your reach.

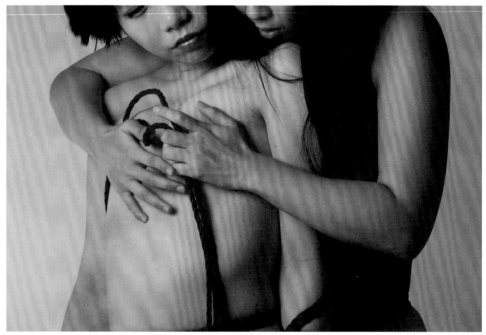

Press up against the Rope Bottom. Use your chest to press into her back, and feel each other's breathing. Extend your arm over her shoulder, and use your body temperature to relax her body. Pull back softly to guide her to stretch out her body and limbs.

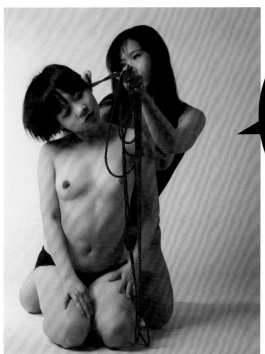

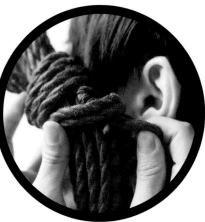

Take advantage of the sound of rope. Hold the bundle of rope up next to her ears. Squeeze the rope bundle to let the Rope Bottom hear the sound of the ropes rubbing each other. Pull on the rope head to undo the rope bundle. Let the rope fall to the floor to make a clear and melodious sound.

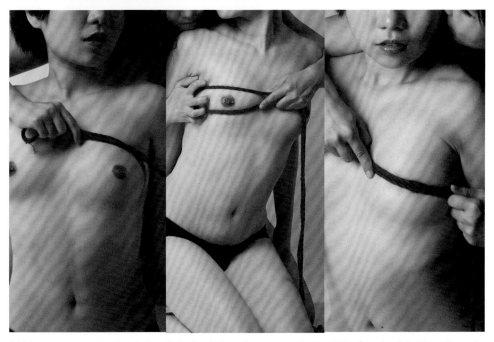

Hold the rope, and press it against the Rope Bottom's skin. Trace the rope across the Rope Bottom's neck and shoulder, pulling on the rope to rub against the rope bottom's skin. You can rub the rope back and forth several times.

Attention: Lark's head knot will get tighter as you pull on it. In the kinbaku play of this chapter, both parties frequently change their postures. Do not use this to hold the wrist for a long time, and do not pull hard on the Rope Bottom's arm. For longer play, use the single column tie as introduced in the next chapter.

Now we introduce the only technique being used in this chapter:

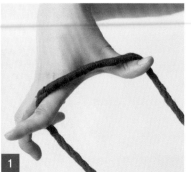

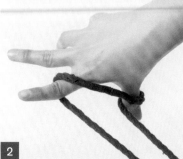

Use thumb and index finger to open up the rope head. Use both fingers to hook the rope from outside to inside.

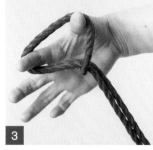

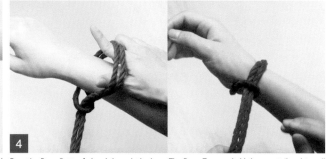

Pull on the rope to form a loop. This is called a lark's head, or cow hitch.

Pass the Rope Bottom's hand through the loop. The Rope Top can hold the rope tail end to pull slightly. Consider wrapping the loop around the Rope Bottom's forearm instead of their wrist.

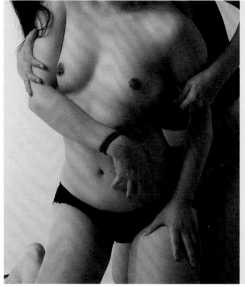

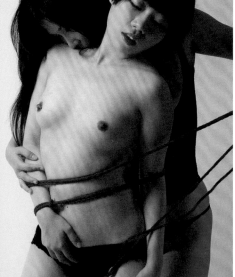

Wrap the rope around the Rope Bottom's body. The speed and force of the second wrap can be different from the first wrap, and the third wrap can be different from the second wrap.

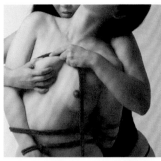 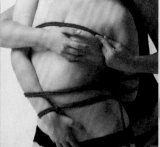 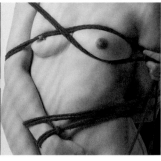

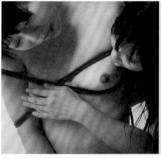 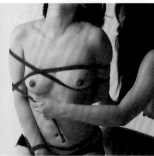

Practice expressing your emotion as you wrap, using your rhythm, force, breathing, expression, and exchanging looks. One wrap can convey closeness and love, but you can also use a different wrap to express a strong longing and desire. It can be used to express joy, or wrath. Let these emotions be conveyed to your partner through your body movement.

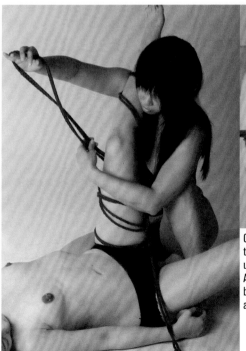 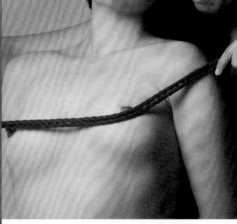

One rope can be used up rather quickly. Now, untie your partner, then wrap her again on different parts of her body. In kinbaku, untying is as important as – or even more important than – tying. As you untie, keep pressing up against her, and let her feel your body temperature along with your affection. Cover her sensitive areas when untying, or you can rub these sensitive areas.

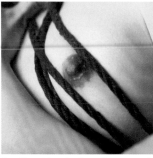

Consider giving the Rope Bottom erotic caresses. You can use the rope to stimulate the sensitive parts of her body; squeeze her breasts to make them stand out; or wrap around her chest or waist.

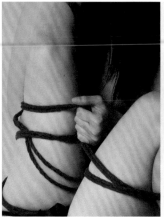

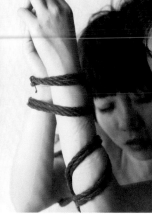

Strive to use minimalistic techniques: no knots, no hooking a rope around another. Only hook a rope around body parts, if following the natural flow of their body. Don't look at the rope. The purpose of doing this is to focus your attention on your partner's body and responses.

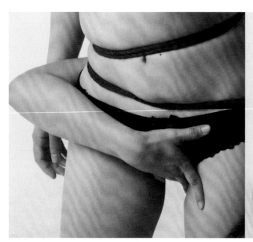

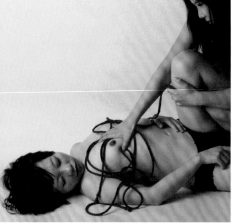

Caress the Rope Bottom's body. Directly touching or use of the rope will cause different sensations. Arms, inner thighs, and ankles are all sensitive areas. You can use a clean rope to press and rub against covered or uncovered private parts based on what you both agreed to in advance. After playing, wash that rope. You may occasionally disrupt the balance of the rope bottom. Let her give up her body, and balance, to you. However, only do so if you can catch her if she falls.

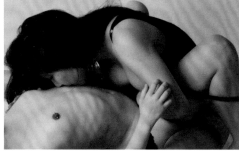

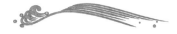

In order not to have your partner feel a break in the flow, or experience a feeling of being abandoned, keep your bodies close to each other as much as possible as you reach for rope or other toys. Even when the Rope Top's upper body is relatively far from the Rope Bottom, it is best for the Rope Top to keep in touch with the Rope Bottom by using the other hand or even the foot. This creates a sense of intimacy.

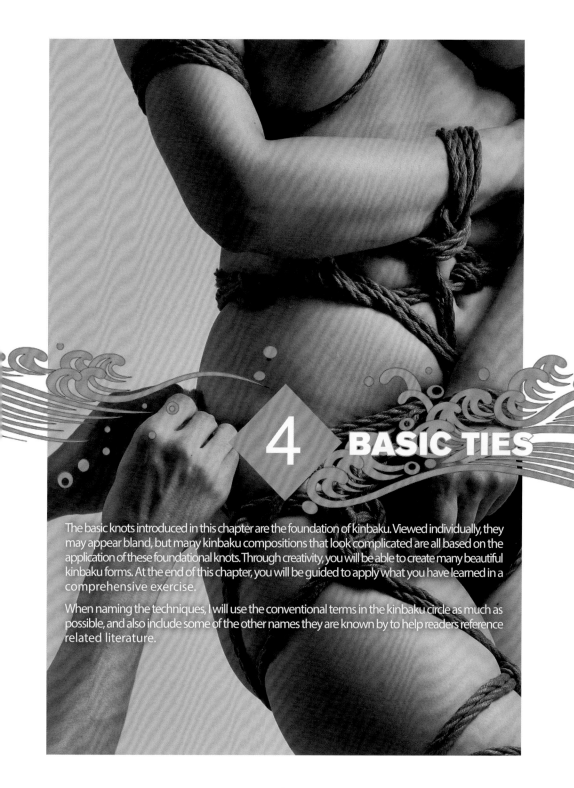

4 BASIC TIES

The basic knots introduced in this chapter are the foundation of kinbaku. Viewed individually, they may appear bland, but many kinbaku compositions that look complicated are all based on the application of these foundational knots. Through creativity, you will be able to create many beautiful kinbaku forms. At the end of this chapter, you will be guided to apply what you have learned in a comprehensive exercise.

When naming the techniques, I will use the conventional terms in the kinbaku circle as much as possible, and also include some of the other names they are known by to help readers reference related literature.

4.1 Single Column Tie

Just as the term implies, this technique can be used to tie column-shaped body parts, such as the arms, thighs, calves, or waist. Although the tie does not look magnificent on its own, it is the foundation of many kinbaku techniques. The single column tie is easy to learn but difficult to master. Even after many years of hard practice of kinbaku, you may not be able to grasp the essentials of many small details of this tie. By observing how smoothly a person executes the single column tie we can judge that person's level of skills.

This tie is suitable to tie the parts of the body where blood vessels and nerves are relatively shallow. Make sure to wrap the tied part several times to form a flat and even surface, and keep a gap between the wraps and the body to allow blood flow. This concrete yet subtle principle of multiple wraps while maintaining gaps is a central tenet of kinbaku.

There are three commonly seen single column ties. The square knot single column tie has relatively few steps, but can be more difficult for a beginner to grasp the appropriate amount of force to be applied. Double square knot single column ties have more steps, but are easier to make the knot firm. Carrick bend 花聯結 single column ties have the advantage of having fewer steps and more firmness, but are difficult to use in situations where the rope wraps need to be relatively tight.

As far as I know, the rope circle in Japan originally did not have a name for this type of tie. Some people use the Japanese term "hon-musubi" [original knot], but that actually refers to the square knot used. Most likely this name was acquired from English terminology.

4.1.1 Single Column Tie

The first type of single column tie is held in place with a square knot. The square knot is one of the most common knots in daily life.

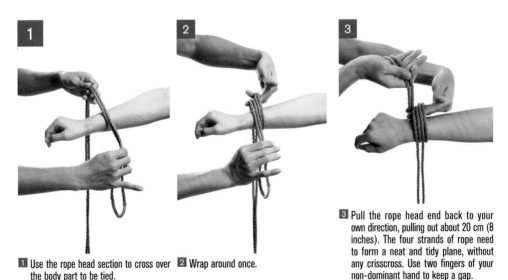

1 Use the rope head section to cross over the body part to be tied.

2 Wrap around once.

3 Pull the rope head end back to your own direction, pulling out about 20 cm (8 inches). The four strands of rope need to form a neat and tidy plane, without any crisscross. Use two fingers of your non-dominant hand to keep a gap.

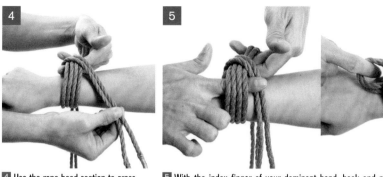

4 Use the rope head section to cross over the four strands of rope.

5 With the index finger of your dominant hand, hook and pull out the rope head. Pay attention that the rope head needs to pass through and under all the four strands of rope.

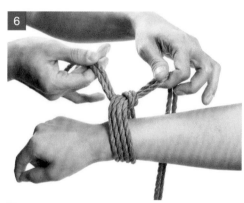

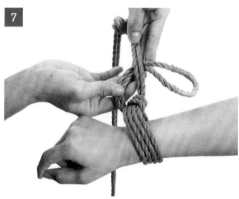

6 Pull out the rope head section. Simultaneously pull the rope head end and the rope tail sections to slightly tighten. This keeps the gap from collapsing, and the four strands of rope on the column body will still forms a neat and tidy plane.

7 Pass the rope head section under the rope tail section.

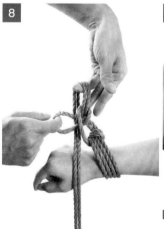

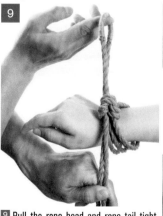

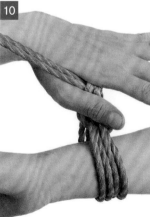

8 Wind the rope head back to where it came from, and pass through the gap formed in Step 7.

9 Pull the rope head and rope tail tight. Pull the rope tail in the direction opposite to what it was in Step 6 and 7. Notice the symmetrical pattern in this picture.

10 Strand by strand, either pull or push the rope until it is tight.

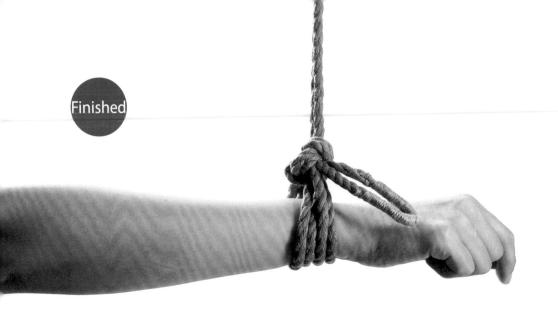

Finished

1. The four strands of rope need to form a leveled and neat plane, wrapping like a belt or "rope ring" to make the rope bottom comfortable.

2. When the rope is being pulled, the knot will not collapse, and the gap is still maintained. The most common reasons that the knot collapses are because the rope tail is being pulled straight (see Figure ❶), causing the knot to slip when the rope is under strain (see Figure ❷). The secret to prevent this from happening is to solidly execute Steps 6, 9, and 10. The direction of pulling the rope head in Step 9 should be opposite to that of Step 6. In Step 10, the knot should be tightened by pushing.

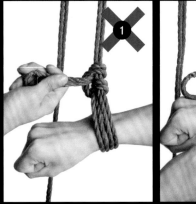

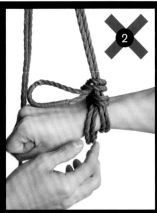

Common mistakes:

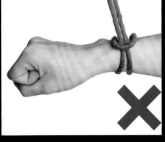

Using a lark's head knot to hook the wrist. The loop will tighten when the rope is pulled, cutting off blood circulation.

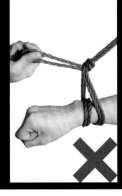

In Step 5, failing to hook all the four strands of rope will cause the loop to tighten when the rope is pulled.

The square knot, reef knot, or "hon-musubi" is not only used to connect ropes, but also used in many ornamentations. If you wind the rope in a wrong direction, you will form a granny knot that is more easily undone.

In the two images below, the upper knots are the square knots. Notice that the red rope on the left side is completely on top of the natural-color rope, and the natural-color rope on the right side is completely under the red rope. Pulling the square knot tight will produce the symmetrical pattern as shown in Step 9. Even if each of the two ropes is pulled to the left and right, the knot will not easily be undone. This is what we hope to see in the square knot single column tie.

The lower knot is the granny knot. The red rope and the natural-color rope are each on top once on both the left side and the right side. Another characteristic of this knot is that pulling it tight will produce a cross-like pattern. The granny knot is more easily undone, so it should be avoided. This principle is also applicable when tying many objects in daily life.

(Special thanks to Mai Maya for help with the material in this section.)

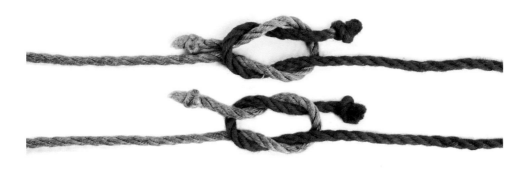

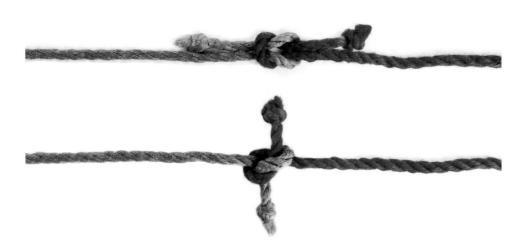

4.1.2 Square Knot Single Column Tie

The square knot single column tie may be completed quickly after much practice, but you need to master appropriate force in order to prevent the knot from slipping. Its firmness also depends on the friction force of the rope you are using. Following is another common technique that adds an additional flat knot. Although there are more steps, it holds more reliably. When tying the double square knot, you need to pay attention to the direction of force applied. If you do not, there is still the possibility of the knot slipping.

Follow Steps 1-6 of the square knot single column tie.

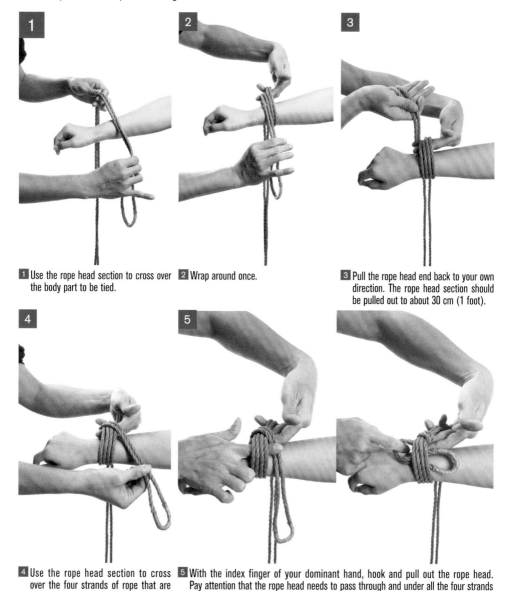

1 Use the rope head section to cross over the body part to be tied.

2 Wrap around once.

3 Pull the rope head end back to your own direction. The rope head section should be pulled out to about 30 cm (1 foot).

4 Use the rope head section to cross over the four strands of rope that are wrapping around the object being tied.

5 With the index finger of your dominant hand, hook and pull out the rope head. Pay attention that the rope head needs to pass through and under all the four strands of rope.

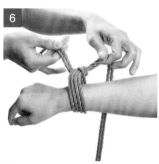

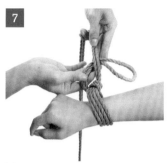

6 Pull out the rope head end and rope tail simultaneously to slightly tighten. By doing so, the gap between the rope and the object being tied will not collapse.

7 Tie a square knot. Make sure to pull the rope tail section towards a direction that is opposite to Step 6. You should see a symmetrically shaped square knot.

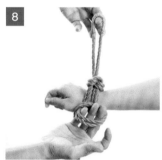

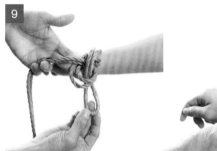

8 Use your non-dominant hand to form a loop with the rope tail section.

9 Thread the rope head through the loop and pull the rope tight. You will see another symmetrical square knot.

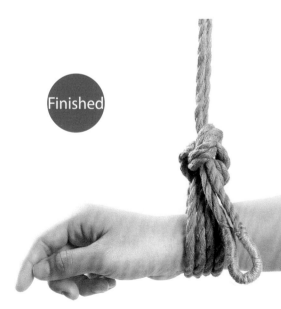

Finished

4.1.3 Carrick Bend Single Column Tie

Using a Carrick bend (also known as the coin knot, sailor knot, and big sheet bend) to tie a single column tie is a recent invention in Europe and America. The application of force is relatively simple, and the knot is firmer. You can quickly tie this knot after much practice, and the knot is suitable for smooth rope. When tying wrists and ankles, there should be some gap between the rope wrap and the body. In such cases, the Carrick bend single column tie is an ideal choice. When tying the hip or other areas where the rope needs to be tight, using a single column tie that primarily uses square knots is encouraged.

In 2010, the American bakushi Topologist modified the Portuguese-style bowline and the French-style bowline to explain the tie in this section. It became named the Somerville bowline. Later, Wykd Dave and others discovered that the knot was in fact the Carrick bend, which has existed for a long time. Therefore, this book uses the original name.

Follow Steps 1-3 of the square knot single column tie.

1 Use the rope head to cross over the body part to be tied, from top to bottom.

2 Wrap around once.

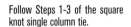

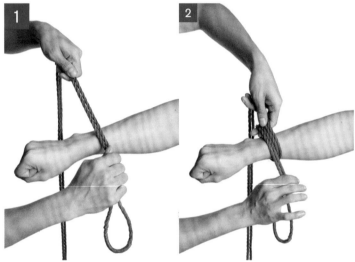

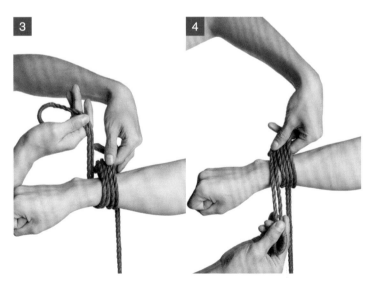

3 Pull the rope head end back to your own direction. Maintain the length to about 30 cm (1 foot).

4 Place the rope head section in parallel to the four strands of rope that are wrapped around the object being tied, and press with the thumb of your non-dominant hand.

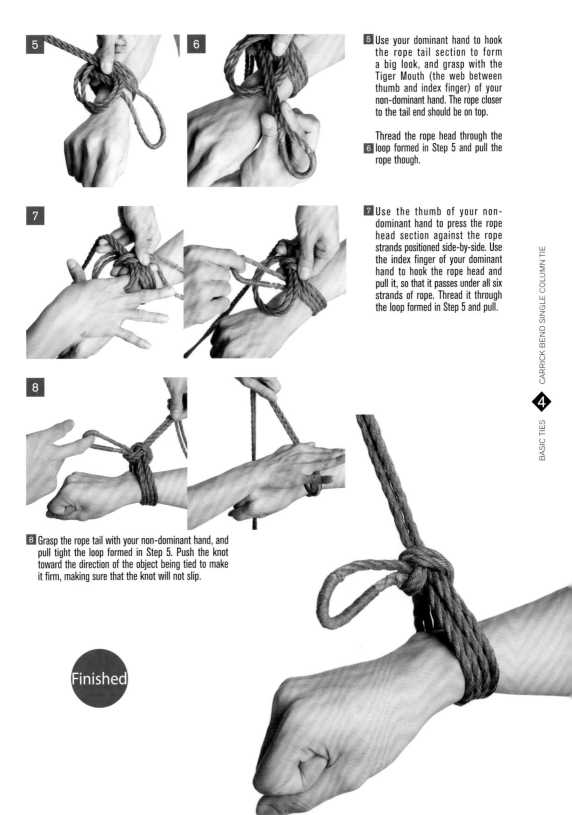

5 Use your dominant hand to hook the rope tail section to form a big look, and grasp with the Tiger Mouth (the web between thumb and index finger) of your non-dominant hand. The rope closer to the tail end should be on top.

6 Thread the rope head through the loop formed in Step 5 and pull the rope though.

7 Use the thumb of your non-dominant hand to press the rope head section against the rope strands positioned side-by-side. Use the index finger of your dominant hand to hook the rope head and pull it, so that it passes under all six strands of rope. Thread it through the loop formed in Step 5 and pull.

8 Grasp the rope tail with your non-dominant hand, and pull tight the loop formed in Step 5. Push the knot toward the direction of the object being tied to make it firm, making sure that the knot will not slip.

Finished

4.2 Double Column Tie

As its name suggests, this tie can be used to tie two column-like objects arranged in parallel; both hands, thighs, calves, or any combination of columns. There are many techniques of double column tie, but here I show a simple method that is similar to the double square knot single column tie.

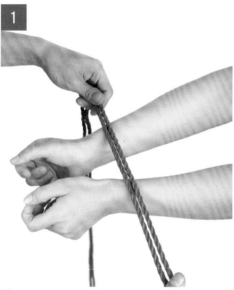

1 Use the rope head to cross over the body parts to be tied, from top to bottom.

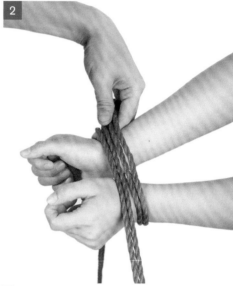

2 Wrap around once.

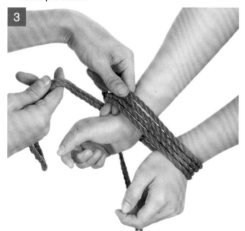

3 Pull the rope head end back towards you. Arrange the four strands of rope to form a neat and tidy plane. The rope head should be pulled out 30-35 cm (12-14 inches). At the same time, a 5-8 cm (2-3 inch) gap should be maintained between the two "columns" being tied. This gap may appear to be too big, but it will be pulled tight in the next few steps.

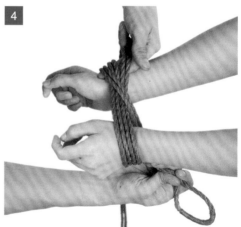

4 Use the rope head section to cross over the four strands of rope that are wrapping around the object being tied.

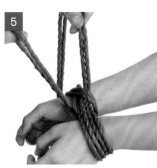

5 Wrap the rope head section around the lowest point.

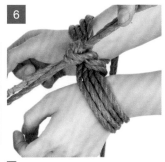

6 Tie a square knot.

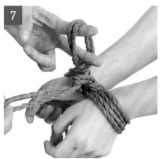

7 With your non-dominant hand, form the tail end of the rope into a loop.

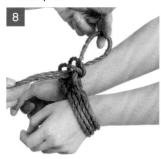

8 Thread the rope head through the loop and pull.

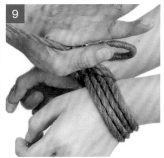

9 Using your non-dominant hand to grasp the rope tail, use your dominant hand to securely push the knot against the objects being tied, making sure that the knot will not slip.

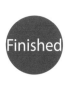

Finished

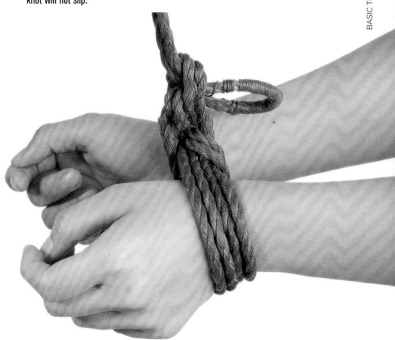

4.3 Half Hitch and Double Half Hitch

After capturing someone's hands and feet with single column or double column ties, you may wish to secure them to a fixed point. Here, we introduce a technique that is often used, even in suspension.

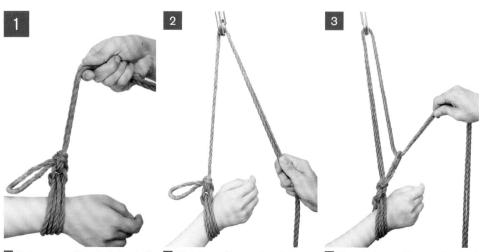

1 Bind someone with a single tie, double column tie, or some other tie with a knot that has a loop that can be hooked.

2 Wind the working section of the rope around the fixed point, whether a carabiner, table leg, bed post, or another sturdy point that can take the load.

3 Thread the working section back through the rope head, and pull.

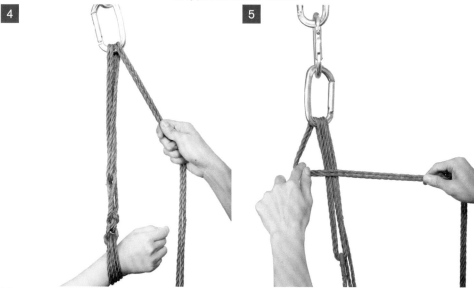

4 Wrap the working section around the fixed point again. You can pull the working end to adjust the distance between the object and the fixed point. Keep the ropes as neat as possible to make it easier to pull the rope.

5 Use your dominant hand to hold onto the working section, and use the non-dominant hand to create an opening.

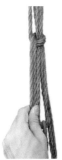

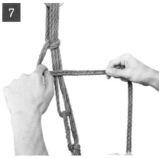

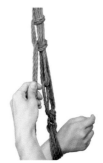

6 Use your dominant hand to push the working section through the opening created in Step 5. Pull the rope down in the direction the rope was going at the end of Step 4. Steps 5 and 6 combined are called a "half hitch" or "hito-musubi."

7 Repeat Steps 5 and 6, forming a second half hitch.

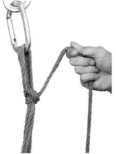

8 Pull the rope upward, causing the two half hitches up against each other. Due to the friction force of the hemp rope, after this step the knot will be fixed, and will not be easily undone.

9

To make the tie look beautiful, it is common to use up the rope that is left over. One method is to thread through the rope head again, and form several half hitches. When about 30 cm (1 foot) of rope is left, wrap it around the weight-supporting rope, and push the rope tail into a crack to jam it in place.

Finished

For those doing suspension, be mindful of safety. After Step 8, please form extra half hitches, tuck the working end through the areas with the tightest friction, and always pull the rope tight. Make sure to use rope and fixed points that are appropriate for suspension.

4.4 Various Styles of Frictions

This section will introduce three techniques that are often used, when ropes cross each other, to lock the rope in place and prevent sliding. These allow kinbaku ties to be divided into independent, smaller pieces. It also has the effect of making the tie look beautiful. The terminology of these frictions are made up by the author. Since the first two techniques only rely on the rope's friction force to temporarily secure the rope, I refer to them using the term "friction" instead of the term "knot."

4.4.1 Figure 8 Friction

The figure 8 friction can be used to secure several strands of rope arranged in parallel. Since kinbaku often needs several strands of rope to be arranged into a belt shape, the figure 8 friction is frequently used. This illustration assumes that the dominant hand is the right hand. If you are left handed, switch left and right in the instructions.

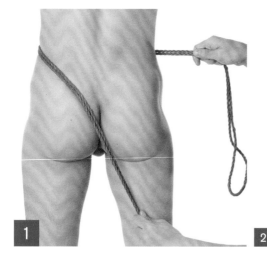

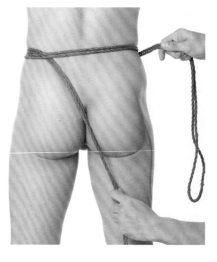

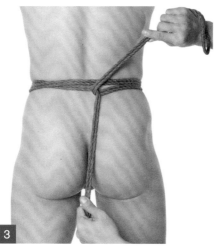

1 Starting from the left side, wrap the rope around the object being tied.

2 Wrap the rope a second time, crossing over the first wrap.

3 Hook the middle rope and turn the line 90 degrees, pulling the rope from right to pointing up.

> In Step 2, the more recent wrap crosses over the older wrap. This temporarily prevents the rope loop from sliding to a narrower part of the body. This is useful when tying the thigh (see Section 6.5) or arm binders (see Section 6.7).

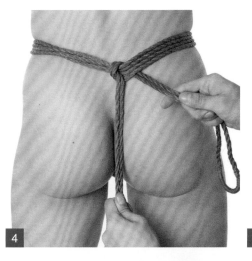

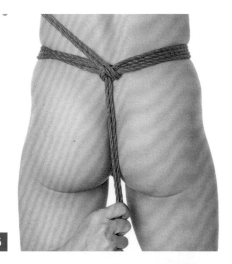

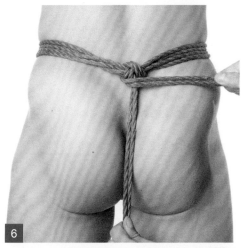

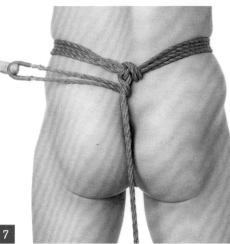

This friction and the next prevent the rope from sliding, but do not completely secure the rope. If there is no tension on the rope, then the friction bend can still be undone. In most cases, both sides of the rope are tied to other parts, so these types of friction will be sufficient.

4 Pass the rope head underneath the parallel strands of rope.

5 Pull the rope upward to the left.

6 Pass the rope head underneath the parallel strands of rope on the other side. Cross over the middle rope, hook it and pull to the right side. Use finger to smooth the wrap, making the parallel strands of rope flat and neat. Adjust the crossing point close to the center. If the rope's working end needs to run to the right, then the figure 8 friction is finished.

7 If the rope's working end needs to run to the left, then you can turn the working end around to hook over the center rope stem.

4.4.2 Cross Friction

Cross friction is often used when two strands of rope cross each other with a fixed crossing point to prevent sliding. The following are two cross friction techniques, showing two reversible sides of the same friction method. This friction is also known as the Munter hitch, Italian hitch, or crossing hitch.

Technique 1.

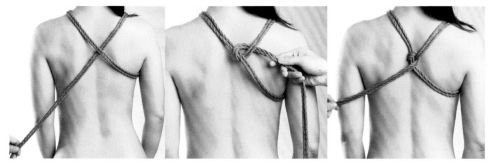

Pass the working section underneath the rope's crossing point, and then proceed as shown.

Technique 2.

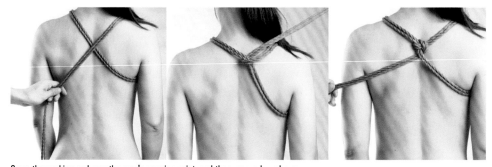

Cross the working end over the rope's crossing point, and then proceed as shown.

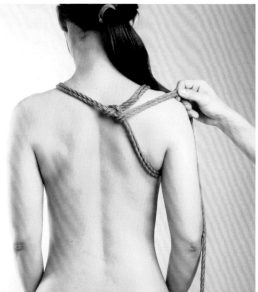

After forming the cross friction, the rope can proceed in the original direction, or may turn back in the opposite direction.

4.4.3 Twisted Cross Friction

The knot formed by the twisted cross friction is bigger than the cross friction, but the rope only needs to be pulled once, and the working end does not need to completely pass underneath the crossed rope. The chance of the crossed rope loosening and falling off is relatively small. This knot is suitable when the working end needs to intersect a relatively taut strand of rope.

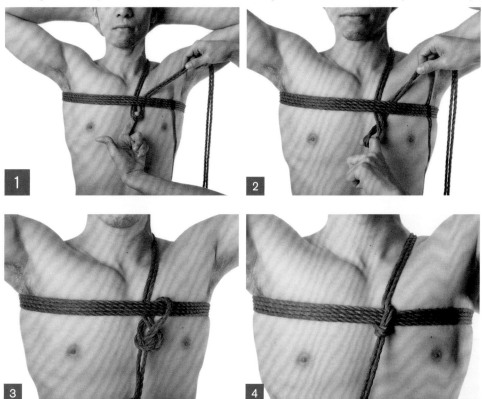

1 Pull out a small section of the working end from underneath the rope being intersected.

2 Twist to form a loop.

3 Pass the working end through the loop formed in the previous step.

4 Pull tight.

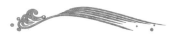

4.5 Connecting Ropes

As previously stated, modern Japanese kinbaku uses ropes between 3.7 to 4 meters (12-13 feet) after they have been folded in half. After the rope is used up, the rope tail can be connected to the rope head of another piece of rope to continue tying. This section introduces several rope connection methods.

4.5.1 Lark's Head

It is customary in kinbaku to form a knot at each of the two ends of a piece of rope. This allows for quick connections of rope using a lark's head.

Usually it is not desirable to place a rope connecting knot at the front of the body (this is not very aesthetically pleasing), or at a sensitive location of the body, as it can cause pain when force is applied. At such a time, you can use the method in the next section to connect ropes early by attaching one rope to the middle of another rope. Use up the excess rope tail end by winding and tucking it.

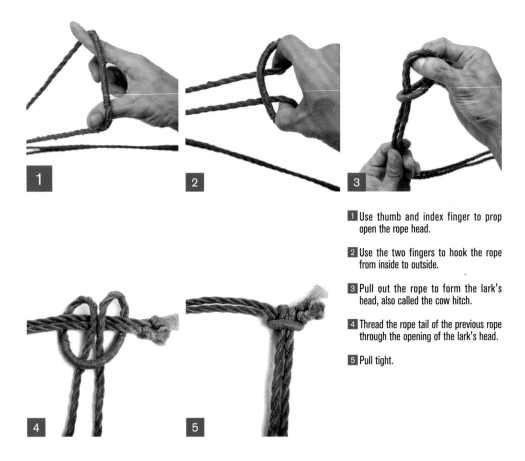

1 Use thumb and index finger to prop open the rope head.

2 Use the two fingers to hook the rope from inside to outside.

3 Pull out the rope to form the lark's head, also called the cow hitch.

4 Thread the rope tail of the previous rope through the opening of the lark's head.

5 Pull tight.

If the two strands of the rope tail are not of equal length, then you can attach the Lark's head around both ropes, then wind back the longer rope tail strand, and push it between the two rope strands to hold it in place.

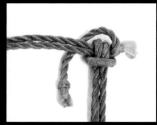 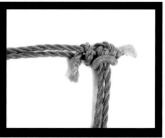

4.5.2 Square Knot

When the previous rope has not been used all the way up to its rope tail but you want to attach the next rope ahead of time, you can use this technique. Those who do not have knots on their rope tails may also prefer to use this method to connect ropes.

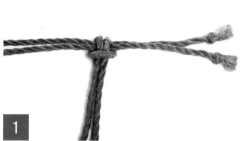

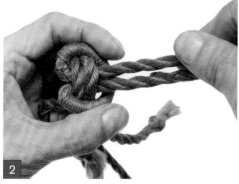

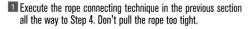

1 Execute the rope connecting technique in the previous section all the way to Step 4. Don't pull the rope too tight.

2 Partially open the lark's head knot, causing the original rope to fold back on itself.

3 Pull tight, so that the lark's head becomes a modified square knot.

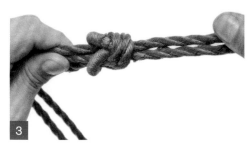

(!) Attention: This method is only suitable for hemp and other ropes with rough surfaces. When using rope with smooth surfaces (e.g., nylon rope), a square knot can easily be pulled back to form a lark's head, and then slip to become undone. The next section will introduce the sheet bend that is suitable for smooth rope.

4.5.3 Sheet Bend

When using nylon rope or other ropes with a smooth surface, you can use the traditional sheet bend by following these four steps as illustrated.

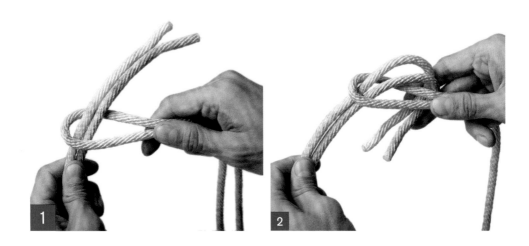

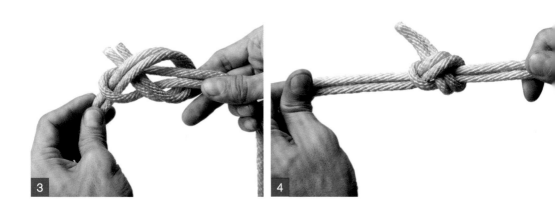

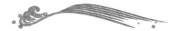

4.6 Lock Stitch Crocheting

The lock stitch technique can weave the rope into a relatively wide flat surface, and is also often used to use up excess rope at the conclusion of a kinbaku tie. It is referred to as the "chain stitch" in crochet, and in Japanese is referred to as "kusariami."

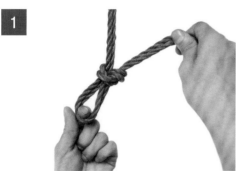

1 Make a slipknot to form a first loop. Alternatively, use the first step of the twisted cross knot to form the first loop.

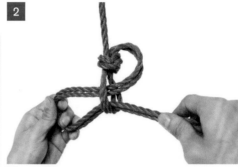

2 Thread the working section through the loop formed in the previous step, and form the next loop.

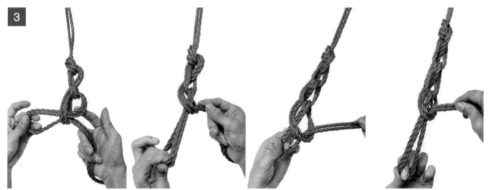

3 Repeat Step 2. Every time you thread the rope to form a loop, pull on the rope to make the knot snug, until the lock stitch reaches the length you want.

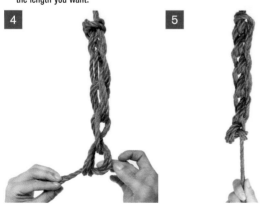

4 Finally pull the working section completely through the loop, and pull tight.

5 When undoing the knot, pull out the working section of the last loop. The rest of the lock stitch can be undone by one pull of the rope to the end.

LOCK STITCH CROCHETING

BASIC TIES

4

4.7 Comprehensive Exercise: Improvisation

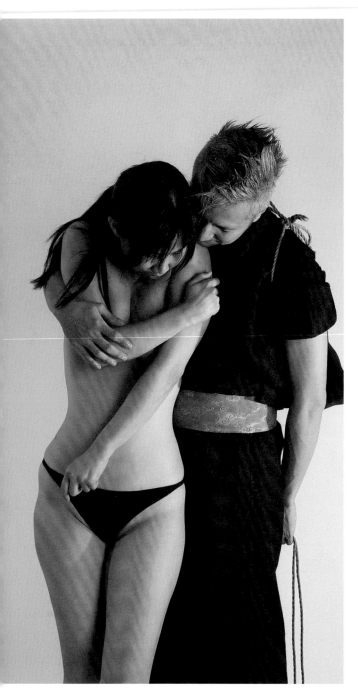

The techniques mentioned in this chapter have already covered the several basic principles of Japanese kinbaku: wrap rope around the parts of body to form flat and neat loops; use ties that are not easily undone to maintain the gap between rope and body; and use techniques such as frictions to partially affix ropes in place. The whole body tie is made up of independent, smaller unit modules.

We will go into safety in the next chapter, and look at common kinbaku ties in Chapter 6. However, as stated in Chapter 1 of this book, a kinbaku teacher can only teach general principles. Those ties that are not in agreement with the general principles are probably not proper, but as to what are the proper things to do, it really depends on individual needs, situations, and creativities. In different situations, the purposes of kinbaku are different. Every Rope Bottom has their own individual preferences. Every Rope Bottom's body is naturally unique. The Rope Top must adapt themselves to changing conditions. Therefore, kinbaku always contains an element of improvisation.

We will demonstrate a kinbaku improvisation exercise in this chapter: starting from an arbitrary part of a body, weave patterns at will on the rope bottom's body. The goal is for readers to discover from this type of exercise how to follow the rope bottom's body type to flexibly bring into play the various techniques they have learned from this chapter, and to adjust immediately as situations develop.

This exercise is inspired by nawashi Pedro Diniz Reis. As he once said, "kinbaku can be like Jazz music, in that every performance is different."

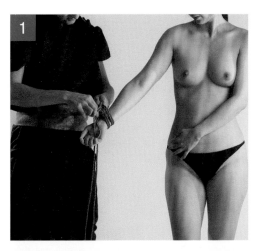

1 Start from single column tie on the right hand.

2 Wrap around the body. Since you may intend to create a relatively solid feel, wrap an extra round to form a loop.

3 At the back, affix the rope in place with a figure 8 friction, change to another direction and wind the rope to the front. When crossing the rope strands, use a cross friction to affix the rope in place.

4 Follow the flow of the rope to wrap once around the waist, and affix the rope with a cross friction when the rope strands cross each other. The rope is about to be used up, so connect ropes at this location.

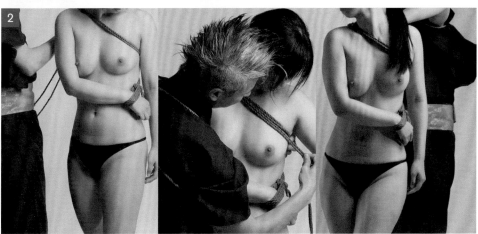

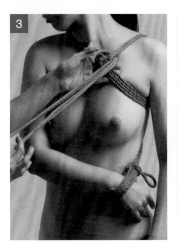

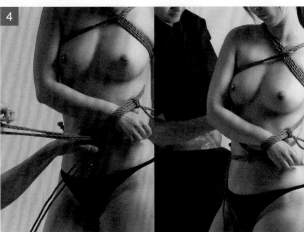

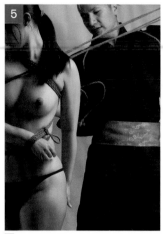
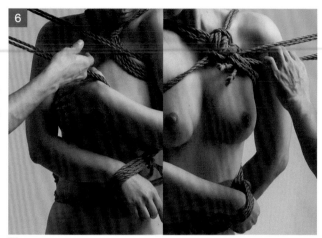

5 Wind the rope to the back. Use a cross friction to hold the crossed ropes in place.

6 From under the armpit, return to the front. Hook the rope's crossing point at the left chest. Wrap the rope around the point several times to form a rose-like shape.

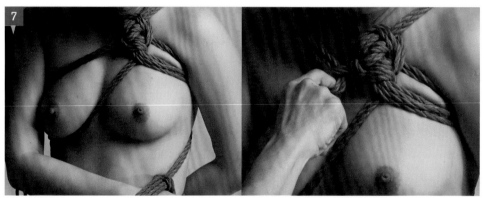

7 Since you may intend to pull the chest rope tight, wind the rope from the other direction, crossing the rope at the chest.

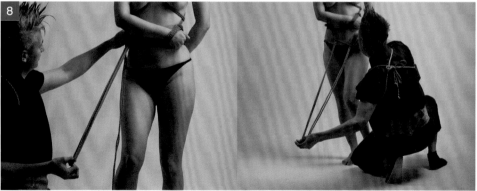

8 Wrap the rope around the lower body. Each time a line crosses another, use a friction of your choosing.

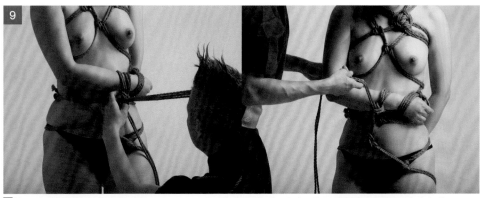

9 If you feel that the arm looks insubstantial, you can use techniques like the single column tie to form a loop around the forearm.

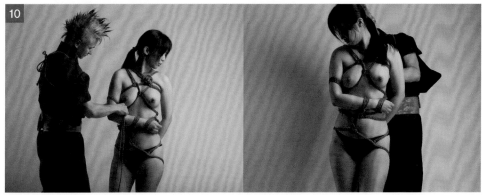

10 Form another loop around the upper arm, winding the rope to the back. It is time to use up the rope that is left over.

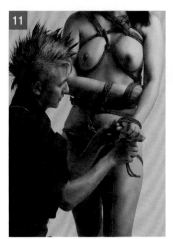

11 Take another piece of rope to start again. Form a single column tie on the left wrist.

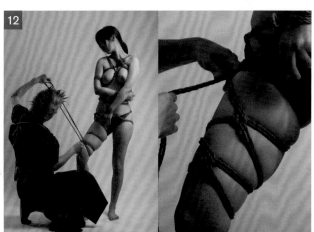

12 Try some decoration on the lower body, winding the rope around the lower body and the thigh. Each time the rope crosses itself, use a friction technique.

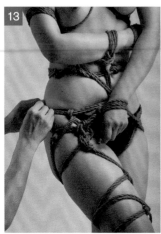

13 Wind the rope to return to the vicinity of the hip. Hook around a previous rope. This may look complex, but it is only a repeated application of the cross friction. Tie or tuck the rope tails to finish.

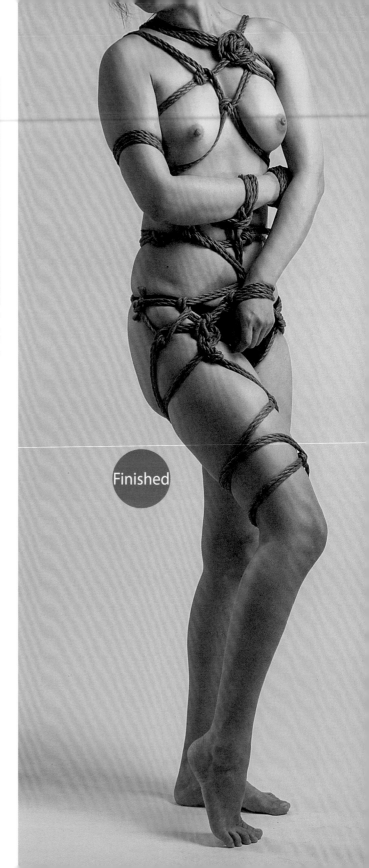

Finished

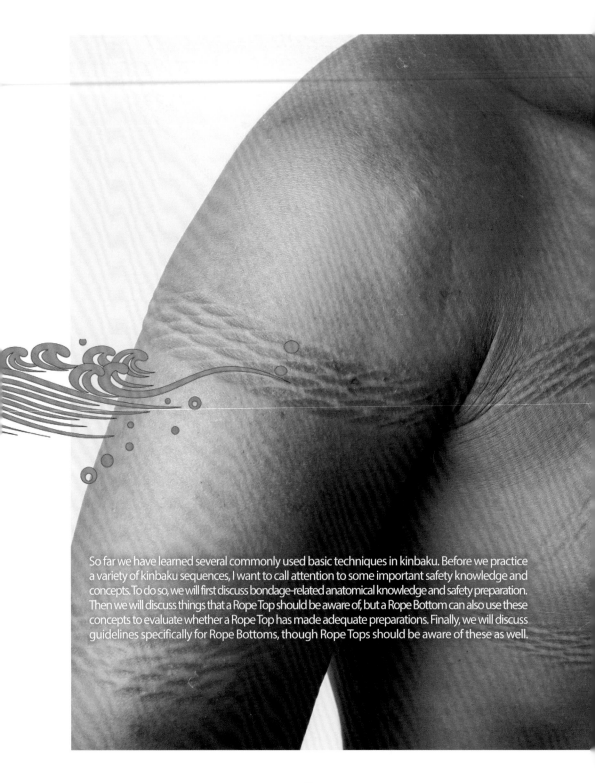

So far we have learned several commonly used basic techniques in kinbaku. Before we practice a variety of kinbaku sequences, I want to call attention to some important safety knowledge and concepts. To do so, we will first discuss bondage-related anatomical knowledge and safety preparation. Then we will discuss things that a Rope Top should be aware of, but a Rope Bottom can also use these concepts to evaluate whether a Rope Top has made adequate preparations. Finally, we will discuss guidelines specifically for Rope Bottoms, though Rope Tops should be aware of these as well.

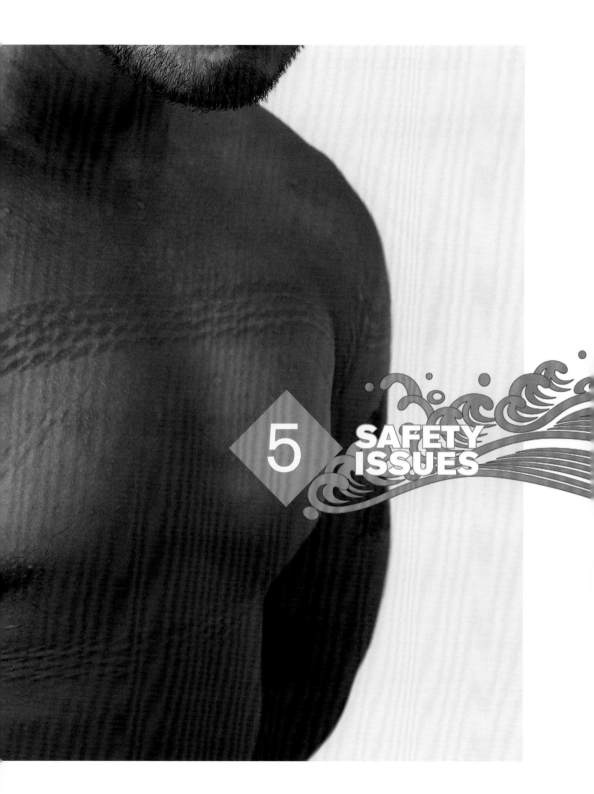

5 SAFETY ISSUES

5.1 Selection of the Body Parts to Tie

Which parts of the body can be tied and which cannot? The general principle is to tie the parts of the body with thick muscles or that are sturdy. Avoid the parts where nerves and blood vessels are relatively shallow. Tie the parts of the body protected by the ribs or the hip bone, and avoid the internal organs.

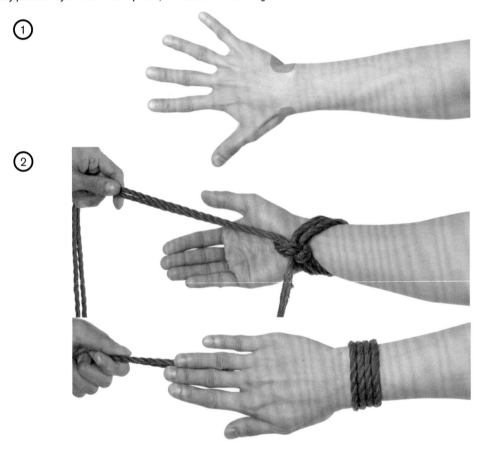

Around the wrist, where the radial and ulna bones join the wrist, the groove on the inside of the wrist is relatively fragile (Figure ①). When tying the wrist, you should adjust the rope to the position shown in Figure ② to avoid the shallow blood vessels. This allows the outer sides of the wrist to bear the force. This position also allows the rope bottom to grab the robe, and use their own grip to reduce some load.

On the arm, the outside of the elbow is fragile, and the inside has relatively shallow nerves and blood vessels. Therefore, the rope should, as much as possible, be tied to the upper arm or the forearm (Figure③). The armpit is the passage where the nerves connect to the arm from the torso, so if it is directly constricted (Figure ④), the rope bottom will quickly feel numbness.

③

④

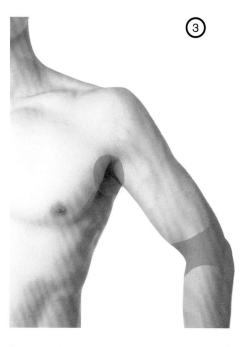

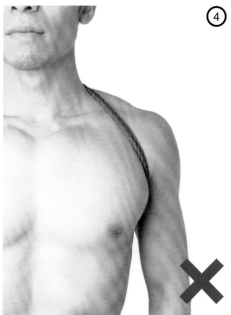

The situation for the leg is similar. The red areas in Figure ⑤ should be avoided. Around the ankle, the single column tie should be wide, and adjusted to avoid the lateral tip (Figure ⑥). This position pulls on the lower leg instead of the foot itself.

⑤   ⑥

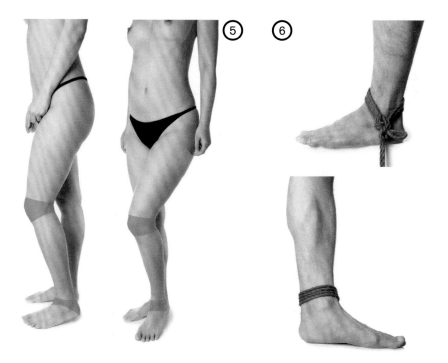

When tying the waist and hip areas, bind the relatively narrower hip area (Figure ⑦), so that the rope is less likely to become loose. However, for suspension or other situations that bear relatively larger forces, most rope bottoms feel that it is more comfortable to tie the rope around the hip bones (Figure ⑧). The hip bones are very strong, and tying here can lower the body's center of gravity while protecting internal organs. For inversions, where the feet are above the head, the position in Figure ⑦ is usually better to hold position around the hip bones and not slip.

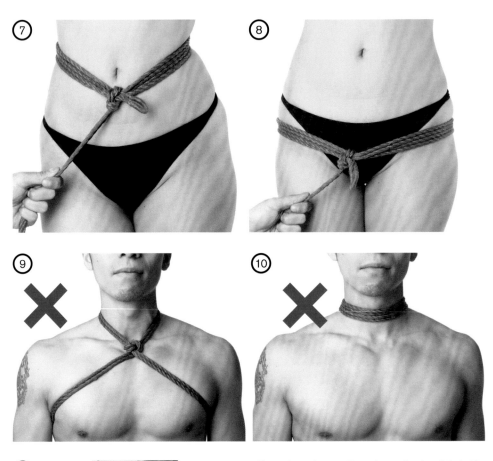

The neck area has carotid arteries passing through both sides, and the windpipe in the middle. This is a very dangerous region to work with. Rope at both sides of the neck can easily compress the carotid arteries (Figure ⑨), and the knot in the middle may impede breathing. The tie in Figure ⑩ is even more dangerous. We suggest you avoid the area around the neck (Figure ⑪).

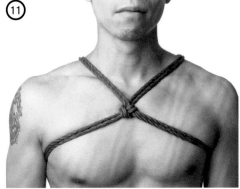

There are those who believe that asphyxiation may enhance sexual pleasure. However, breath-play-related sex games are all highly dangerous. Compressing the carotid artery can cause a lack of oxygen to the brain, leading to fainting in about ten seconds, and further compounded by an innate difference among individual persons; the controllable range of safety is extremely small. Therefore, breath play is an activity akin to walking a tight rope. Even for those SM players who regard themselves as highly experienced, the possibility of careless accidents is still there. It can be said that death due to asphyxiation is the most frequent occurrence of fatal accidents within the SM circle. This book strongly suggests that the readers should refrain from experimenting with play that is related to breath control and asphyxia, and that kinbaku play should avoid areas around the neck, throat, and cervical vertebra as much as possible.

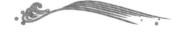

5.2 Nerve Compression

It is a common misconception that watching if see if a llimb turns purple is a sufficient indicator of whether or not circulation is being blocked. This is a relatively unreliable basis of judgment. Color change is more discernable on those with light skin than dark. Compared to blood flow blockage, nerve compression is currently thought to be more dangerous, deserving quicker response. Kinbaku play that follows safety principles is not likely to completely cut off blood circulation. The key is to stay attentive, check on a Rope Bottom's ability to move their hands, change positions, and be okay untying without worry. Troubleshooting and trust can go a long way.

There is an enormous variation in how fast an injury may occur, and the time it takes for different people to recover. For some, just a few minutes can cause issues, with slight symptoms going away quickly. There are also people who have done suspensions that have lost use of their arm for several weeks or months. In order to avoid nerve injury, the Rope Top needs to have a basic understanding of the locations of the nerves and the symptoms of injuries. It is also important for the Rope Bottom to recognize their own body's sensations, and inform the Rope Top of signs and symptoms in a timely manner.

The first symptom of blood flow blockage and nerve compression is for the Rope Bottom to feel numbness. Obstructed blood circulation often causes a large area (such as the whole hand or arm) to experience numbness or a pins-and-needles prickly feeling, accompanied by swelling and pain. Numbness and a prickly feeling caused by nerve compression is limited to a smaller area (such as half a hand, either the first three fingers or the latter two fingers), and is often accompanied by a lack of strength at the extremity of the body. It can also include a stabbing sensation.

Though uncommon, if the above symptoms occur without leaving the ground, then they are often caused by improper compression of the nerves, and should be dealt with as quickly as possible, or the tie should be undone. Numbness and prickly feeling may occur at a body extremity. For example, when the little finger or the ring finger feels numbness and prickliness, it may be caused by the ulnar nerve of the forearm or the elbow being compressed (see Chapter 7.1.3).

Compression may be directly caused by the rope. For such an occasion, the rope may be loosened, or adjusted to other locations. The compression may also be caused by body posture: for example, when lifting the arm above the head, the brachial plexus under the armpit also shifts, thus shifting the area of concern. Lying down or sitting in the same posture might also cause the compression, with each person having different tolerances. In such a situation you should help the rope bottom to change their position, or conclude the current stage of bondage.

It is up to the Rope Bottom to actively convey such feelings and responses to the Rope Top. Every person's muscle strength, tolerance, and capacity are somewhat different. The bondage posture, degree of tightness, and time duration suitable for one person are not necessarily acceptable to another. A Rope Top must cultivate a degree of intimacy with the Rope Bottom, learn about their body's characteristics and responses, encourage them to share their feelings, and work to identify the ties that are best for both parties. The Rope Bottom is indeed the best teacher.

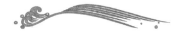

5.3 Instructions for Rope Tops

Rope Tops are encouraged to follow basic etiquette of BDSM communities. Do not touch others without explicit consent, and do not join other's play without invitation. It is inappropriate to assume that just because you have seen someone play in a specific way with someone else, that the person would want to do so with you. If your purpose of play is D/S (domination and submission), you should set a safe word: when the other party says this safe word, the play should stop.

5.3.1 Building the Mental Aspects of Bondage

When meeting your play partner for the first time, spend some time chatting with them and learn about their physical condition: have they been tied up before? How is their flexibility and endurance? Have they been injured? What might be their emotional response under pressure? Depending on their experience, they may or may not be aware of their limits.

Before kinbaku practice, you need to give your partner a general idea about what kind of bondage you are about to do, and mentally prepare them for what is to come, so that it is easier for your rope bottom to cooperate with you later. It is acceptable to reserve some surprises in D/S play, but whatever the situation, the Rope Top should inform the Rope Bottom of possible risks, what type of discomfort may happen in the upcoming bondage, and what rope marks may remain.

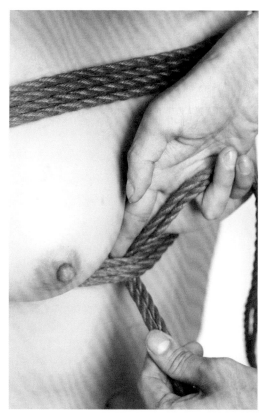

Instead of turning the Rope Bottom back and forth in practice, you should move yourself around the rope bottom to avoid dizziness. When pulling or drawing on the rope next to the Rope Bottom's body, use your own hand to cover the skin in order to prevent scraping and bruising. These show respect for the Rope Bottom. During D/S or other types of play, the aforementioned rules may be relaxed, but you should still avoid unplanned injuries from rope friction.

Constantly pay attention to the Rope Bottom's physical condition, and check in with them. Don't ignore the warning signs they give regarding aches, numbness, and tingling sensations. In the process of bondage, protect the rope bottom: Prevent him or her from outside interruptions that are not preplanned (such as being touched by other people without permission), and administer first aid during sudden emergencies. Do not leave your partner – the rope bottom has entrusted you with their safety.

5.3.2 Location and Equipment

If the temperature is cold, the Rope Bottom's flexibility and endurance will both decrease. Rope Tops can may feel hot due to their own increased activity, which means they may not notice the real temperature in the room.

After being tightly bound, the Rope Bottom may also lose the ability to save themselves during an emergency. The Rope Top is responsible for the protection of his partner. When practicing bondage at an unfamiliar location, keep an eye open for an escape route, or other similar information. Tops are also advised to have some kind of equipment for cutting the rope during an emergency. A commonly used choice is trauma shears (see below). They do not look sharp, but can cut through clothing and rope.

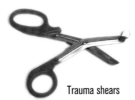

Trauma shears

During partial suspension, or any tie where people are pulling on an overhead point, many people wonder if the rope may break. Though not impossible, new hemp rope is usually sufficient to support many people's body weight. However, once an old rope has experienced wear and tear, Rope Tops must remove that rope from such play. Most suspensions are not supported by only one rope, and every piece of rope is wound back and forth several times.

The most common risk is the suspension point. A suspension point needs to be tied around a strong and secure beam, or drilled into a beam (or into the wall) and bolted on the opposite side. A Rope Top may not know whether the person that put in an anchor point did so proficiently, if load-bearing was taken into consideration when it was installed, or if the anchor point has become worn out. Find this out before playing, testing the point each time, as some things that look like suspension points are not.

Some things that look sturdy are only decorations that cannot bear weight. For example, do not use doors and coat hangers to suspend a person. Implements used for suspension, such as carabiners, can only be used if they are certified specialty equipment for mountaineering or engineering. Many items that look like carabiners are only decorative.

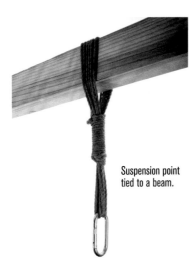

Suspension point
tied to a beam.

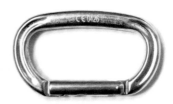

Carabiner used for mountaineering.
It has markings that show the
maximum active load in each of the
horizontal and vertical directions.

5.4 Instructions for Rope Bottoms

Avoid meeting new people in private if they are unknown to you. Rather than establishing a relationship with an individual person alone, it is better to get to know a few friends within the community, thus making it easier to learn about that individual's reputation and skills. Before meeting a stranger, let a friend know where you are going, and check in with them after you are done playing. If you do not check in with this "safe call," that friend can look into it or let authorities know.

Much of the following content is a result of consulting the *Rope Bottom Guide* by the well-known British bondage model and photographer Clover.

5.4.1 Choose a Partner Carefully

Before letting an unfamiliar Rope Top tie you up, use the following tools for evaluation.

How experienced is the rope Top?

Although experience does not necessarily equate to skill level, it is still useful to know. The other party may be brand new. If they are your partner, this can be an opportunity to grow together. If they are not, letting the other party practice on you is a form of generosity and goodwill on your part.

Who has the other party tied with before? What is their reputation in the community?

This is the function of an active and trustworthy BDSM community. Get in touch with the local social gatherings and parties, get involved, and establish a network of support. This is safer than meeting in people in private, and gives you a chance to talk with people who know the Top.

Is the other party knowledgeable about bondage safety?

The Rope Bottom needs to have some basic knowledge, such as what is in this book, in order to evaluate the Rope Top. After talking with the Rope Top, if they did not do their homework as adequately as you, carefully consider whether you can entrust them with your safety.

Does the other party have safety items such as trauma shears?

This is another way to tell if your partner is prepared.

5.4.2 Know Yourself

In addition to possessing basic rope safety knowledge, learn about your own body as much as possible. Press on your arm to find your nerve bundles, figure out which areas are most likely to feel tingly, and which places can endure a fair amount of force. Some people's thigh muscles are relatively strong, while other people will easily have aches and tingly feeling as soon as they raise their limb. Every person's flexibility is somewhat different – Rope Tops need to adjust accordingly.

Does your body have any old injuries? Should some areas be avoided during the bondage? Be aware of your own psychological conditions, and what might make you nervous. Were there any unpleasant experiences in past bondage play? Before being tied up, tell the other party about physical and psychological conditions, as well as your old injuries, so play can be good for everyone. Skilled nawashi can make thoughtful adjustments so that even people with scoliosis can find safe postures. To do so, it is imperative that you inform the other party about your various concerns beforehand.

As discussed in the previous section, blocked blood circulation generally causes numbness and prickly feelings on a relatively larger area, and is often accompanied by a swelling feeling. Nerve compression often happens in a small area, and is accompanied by a lack of strength at the extremity. Some Rope Bottoms can learn to differentiate between these two feelings through experience, informing the Rope Top as soon as they occur, so that the situation can be taken care of immediately. For some ties, such as takate kote (see Chapter 7), holding good posture can also aid in maintaining circulation and reduce the chances of nerve compression. Keeping clear communication going, especially if these issues arise, is key.

Remember to do stretching and warm up before the bondage session in order to reduce the chances of injury. It is not advisable to be tied up while you are on an empty stomach or are hungry. Many models are concerned about their body not looking good, but eating is necessary to have great sessions. Many people mistakenly believe that being tied up is easy, but maintaining even simple postures consumes energy. Suspension requires even more muscular power for support, and even breathing is not as easy as under normal circumstances. Such activities test one's stamina. After one session of suspension, a Rope Bottom can be drenched in sweat.

Bondage, even without taking someone off the ground, may leave rope marks as shown in the picture below. Such marks should disappear within an hour or two. Suspension may leave rope marks in areas being bound by the rope, with long red marks potentially left due to capillary blood vessel rupture in the spaces between ropes. These types of rope marks

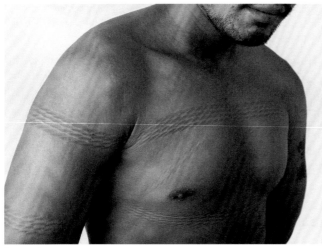

may remain on the body for three or four days, or up to more than one week, depending on one's physique. Compared with nerve injury, rope marks are only a superficial injury that you need not be too worried about. However, if you need to wear short-sleeve clothes within a week, and do not wish people to see the rope marks, then you may need to give up scenes with intense struggling, partial suspension, or full suspension play.

Rope marks.

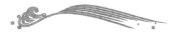

5.4.3 Models and Performance

I want to discuss issues pertaining to photography and performance models, be they professional, part-time, or guest performers. These issues may also arise for others. The reason is because they are the people that will, due to their professional attitude, most likely compromise themselves and do things that are beyond safety limits. However, even if you get paid for your work, you should not ignore your own safety. When your experience signs of discomfort, or discover that the Rope Top has obviously done something wrong, you should inform the photographer and the Rope Top. There is no need for suffering or risking harm, and this can also be a valuable learning opportunity for the Rope Top.

If the photographer or the Rope Top perform acts that are outside the scope of previous agreements, then you should firmly stop everything. Within the photography circle of Taiwan, there is often the bad habit of "coercing the model to give up more," an issue that also happens in the West. This sort of conduct may have an additional serious consequence in bondage photography: If photographers and Rope Tops do not keep their promises, they are likely not treat your safety as a priority. Your consent, and pre-agreed limits, should always be respected – no matter who you are. For models specifically, make sure you have a way to stop the shoot, and if working with a new person, it is best to be accompanied by a trustworthy agent or friend.

Do not think that if you cannot achieve a certain act, or cannot endure a certain tie, that not doing the show they had in mind is your fault. A good nawashi should be able to coordinate with their model, and develop bondage acts that are suitable for both parties. A good performance should not place all the burden on the model, and use only the suffering of the model to entertain the audience. Pain and suffering should only be embellishment. Doing the same extreme tie from start to finish will, on the contrary, only numb and desensitize the audience. Suffering must be "worth it;" the more pain and suffering, the bigger theatrical effect should come as a result. Otherwise, the pain and suffering will only be wastefully squandered.

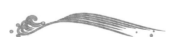

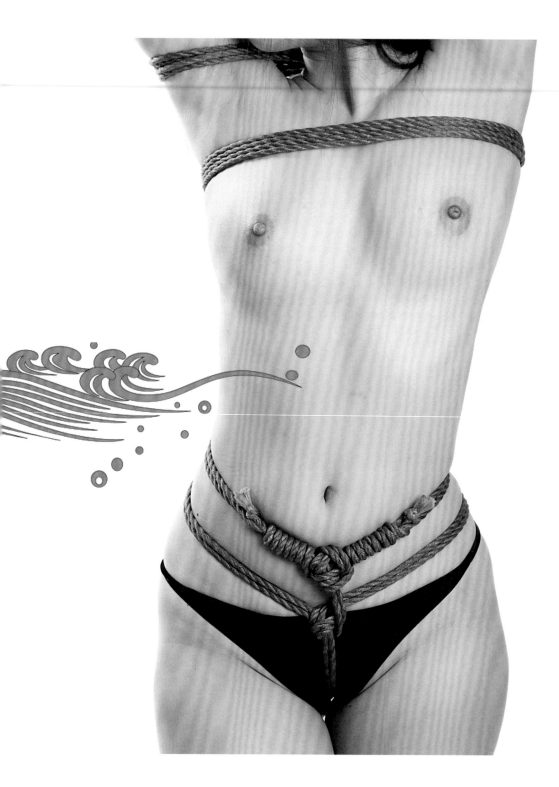

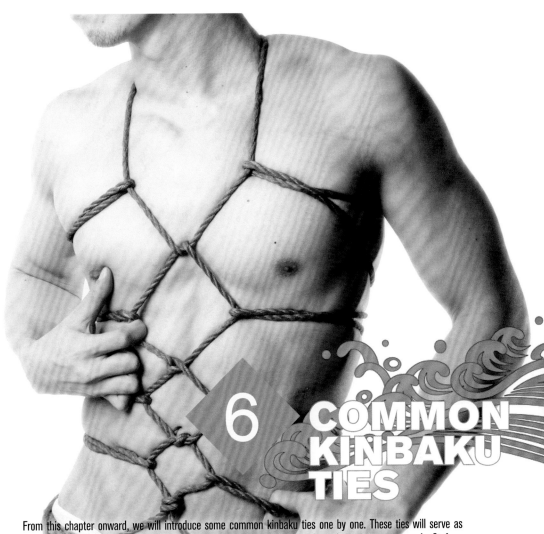

6 COMMON KINBAKU TIES

From this chapter onward, we will introduce some common kinbaku ties one by one. These ties will serve as a reference, and readers must explore their own desires in play based on their circumstances. As Stefano Laforgia might say, kinbaku is like a salad bar, as not every course fits your appetite. We hope that readers can select options suitable for them from the menu of possibilities in this book, and arrange them to make a delicious meal.

6.1 Hands Behind the Head Tie

"Hands behind the head tie" means placing both hands on the back of the head. The name may originate from the nawashi Arisue Go. There are also many other names such as "te-age shibari" [hands-raised tie], or "koutou ryote shibari" [both hands behind the head tie]. This section will first introduce a version that only needs one piece of rope to finish, and is suitable for playing erotic games. Then we will learn a variation that has more stability for holding the position longer.

6.1.1 Crotch Rope Version

1 Begin by tying the rope bottom's hands with double column tie.

2 Lift the Rope Bottom's hands, and pull them down behind their head. The tie will tighten due to the posture, so step 1 should have a gap between the hands.

3 Wind the rope around the Rope Bottom's crotch, then proceed to the right to wind the rope around the waist.

4 Hook the rope back around the rope stem at the center.

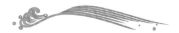

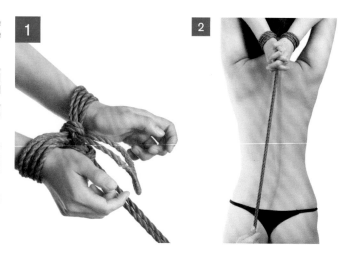

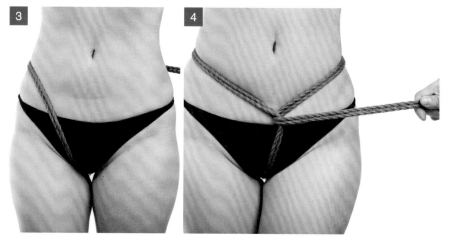

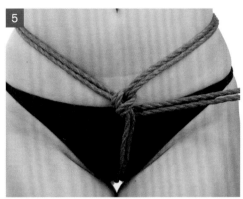

5 Affix with a figure 8 friction.

6 The leftover rope can be used to make rope rings around the waist as in steps 4-5. Pull tight and finish the winding, or make other embellishment according to your creative ideas.

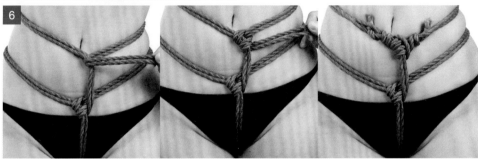

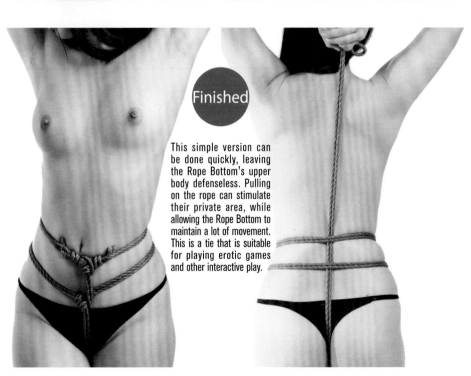

Finished

This simple version can be done quickly, leaving the Rope Bottom's upper body defenseless. Pulling on the rope can stimulate their private area, while allowing the Rope Bottom to maintain a lot of movement. This is a tie that is suitable for playing erotic games and other interactive play.

6.1.2 Affixed Upper Arm Variation

The previous tie allows for easy escape. Just a little struggle will bring both arms to the front of the body. This variation is more restrictive, affixing the Rope Bottom's upper arms as well.

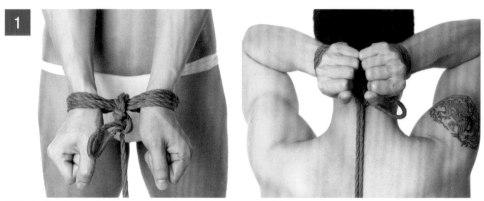

1 Tie the Rope Bottom's hands with double column tie, raise them, and pull them to the back.

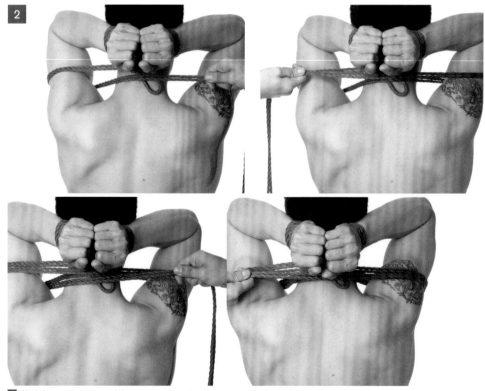

2 Wind the rope twice around the upper arm, keeping the ropes on the back of the neck.

3

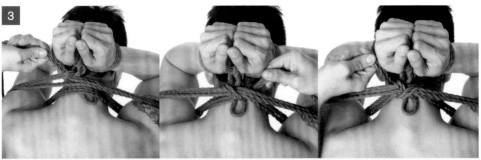

3 Grab all eight strands of rope, and affix them with a figure 8 friction.

4

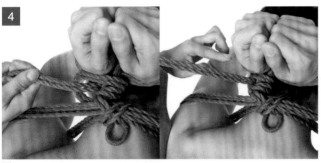

4 Form a half hitch, pulling tight to end the tie.

5

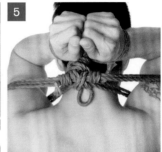

5 Wrap the leftover rope around available areas.

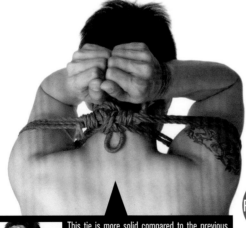

This tie is more solid compared to the previous version. However, it can compress the upper arm and may not be tolerated for long. If you anticipate that the bottom will be lying down, leave much more room in step 1, and adjust their palms to a crossed posture. This will be more comfortable and last longer.

Finished

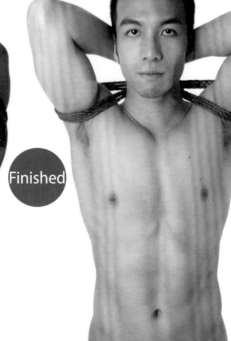

6.1.3 Additional Variations

Starting from the basic versions shown in the previous two sections, you can make all kinds of variations based on your creative ideas.

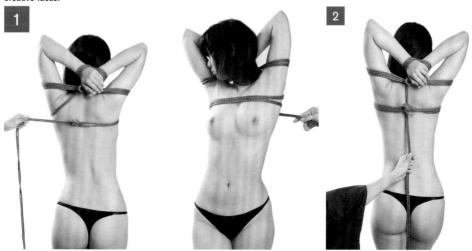

1 After step 4 of the previous section, tie off, and wind the rope twice around the upper body.

2 Use figure 8 friction to affix the rope at the back.

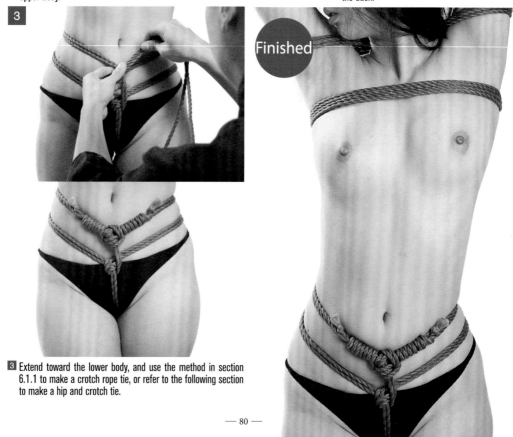

3 Extend toward the lower body, and use the method in section 6.1.1 to make a crotch rope tie, or refer to the following section to make a hip and crotch tie.

Finished

6.2 Hip and Crotch Tie

This section will introduce several methods to tie the lower part of the body. They can be used for sex games, and some can be used to provide support for partial and full suspension. In the West, this type of bondage is referred to as a hip harness. In Japan, each element of the tie is separately called a waist rope and crotch rope. "Hip and crotch tie" 腰胯縛 is a Chinese term that the author came up with himself. As discussed in Chapter 5.1, when the rope is tied to the waist, it is harder to loosen, making it suitable to hold onto during sex play. Meanwhile, the hip is more capable of bearing force in challenging poses. Choose which is best for you based on your circumstance.

6.2.1 Simple Version for Women

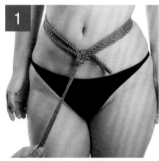

1 Form a single column tie at the waist or hip area. This example shows tying the waist area.

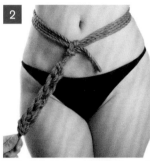

2 Use lock stitch crocheting to form a flat section 30 cm (1 foot) in length.

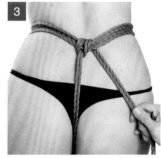

3 Pass the crocheted rope section through the crotch, hook the waist rope, and form a cross friction.

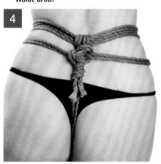

4 Wind the leftover rope around the body to use it up, forming some embellishment.

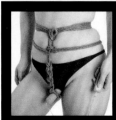

The lock stitch crochet through the crotch can be used to hold various sex toys.

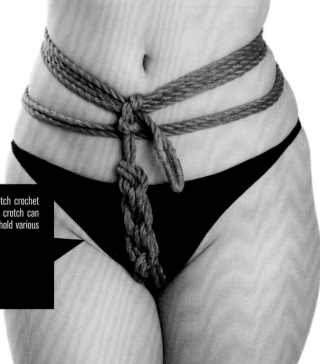

6.2.2 Simple Version for Men

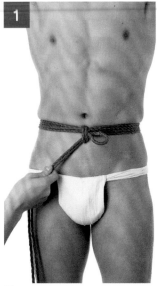

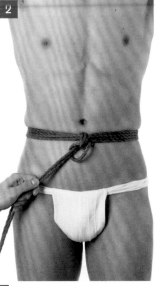

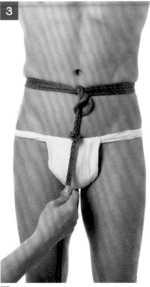

1 Form a single column tie at the waist or hip area. This example shows tying the waist area.

2 You can pass the rope tail end through the rope head, in order to prevent it from coming loose if there will be stress on the rope. Otherwise, this step can be skipped.

3 Form an overhand knot above the penis.

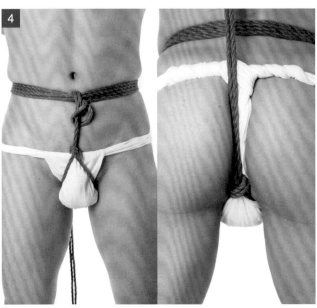

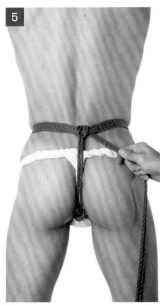

4 Split the rope around the genitals. Form another overhand knot behind the scrotum, at the perineum area.

5 Bring the rope up, hook the waist rope, and form a cross friction.

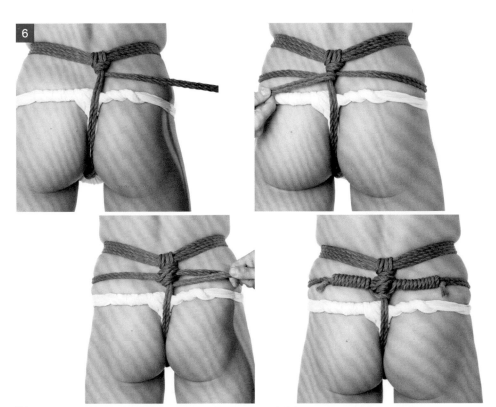

6 Wind the leftover rope around the body to use it up, forming some embellishment.

Finished

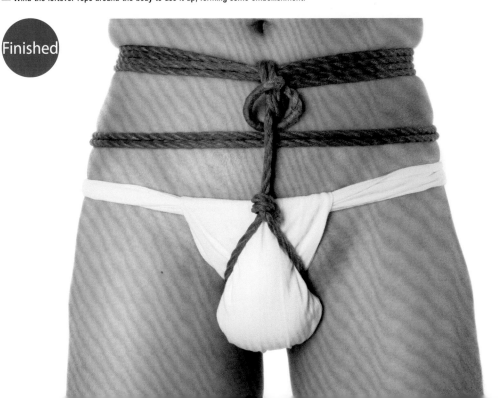

6.2.3 Akechi/Kanna Style Hip and Crotch Tie

This is a style of hip and crotch tie taught by Kanna, and can be traced to the nawashi Akechi Denki. Resembling a rock-climbing sling, it is sometimes used for suspension bondage. It can also be used for embellishment and ornamentation.

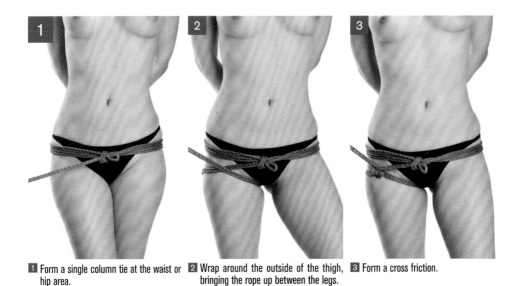

1 Form a single column tie at the waist or hip area.

2 Wrap around the outside of the thigh, bringing the rope up between the legs.

3 Form a cross friction.

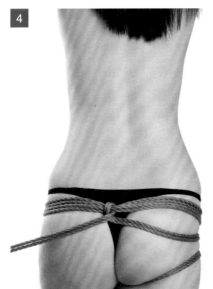

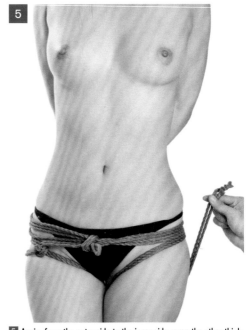

4 Hook the hip (or waist) rope at the center back.

5 Again, from the outer side to the inner side, wrap the other thigh.

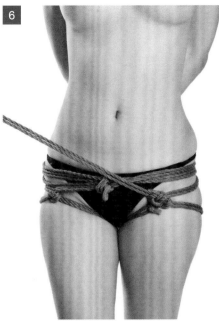

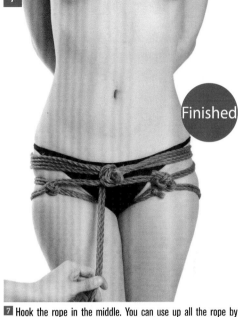

Finished

6 Form a cross friction.

7 Hook the rope in the middle. You can use up all the rope by referring to the several methods described below.

The purpose of the rope rings around the thighs is to prevent the hip from sliding upwards, and distribute pressure. Even with these wraps, the main area that bears the force should will still be the hip area.

Variation 1:
Tie the waist rope, then tie the hip rope, and finally wrap the thighs. This tie is used by nawashi Hajime Kinoko. Since both the waist and hip areas have support, this tie is suitable for many suspension postures.

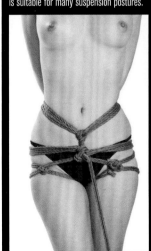

Variation 2:
Use the leftover rope to form a crotch tie.

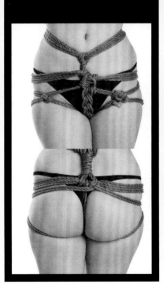

Variation 3:
Wrap around each thigh twice to form the thigh rope rings, in order to ensure comfort.

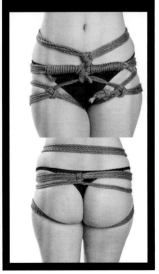

6.3 Pentacle Chest Tie

Chest ties bind the trunk, while allowing both hands to maintain movement. They are common in both the East and West. This version shows a number of embellishments.

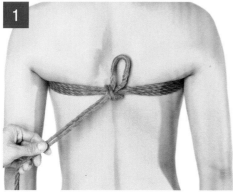

1 Form a single column tie around the Rope Bottom's upper chest area, below the armpits.

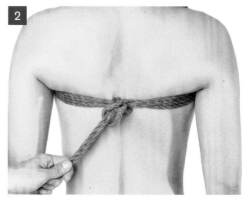

2 For suspension, the rope tail end can pass through the rope head, in order to prevent becoming loose.

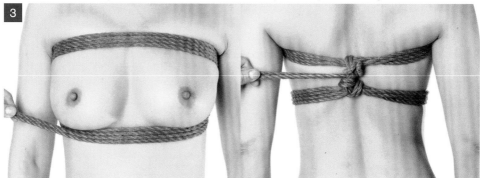

3 Wrap the working section twice around the Rope Bottom's lower chest area, and affix the rope with a figure 8 friction.

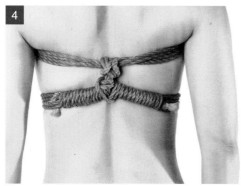

4 Wrap the leftover rope around the rope ring. Tuck the rope head into a gap between ropes.

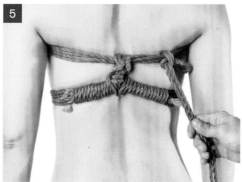

5 Tie a new piece of rope to the upper chest ring near the Rope Bottom's right scapula (shoulder blade), using a half hitch knot.

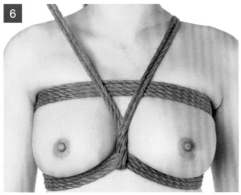

6 Pass the rope over the left shoulder. Hook around the lower rope ring. Pull the rope up slightly before passing the rope under the angled line to reduce sliding of the rope.

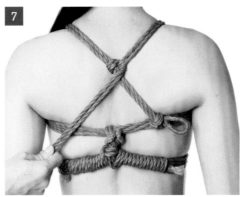

7 Bring the rope over the Rope Bottom's right shoulder. Cross the perpendicular rope and form a cross friction.

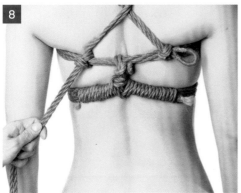

8 Form a twisted cross friction with the upper chest rope ring. This is easier to do than the cross knot since the upper chest rope ring is relatively tight.

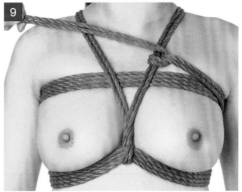

9 Pass the rope under the Rope Bottom's left armpit, and return to the front. Form a cross friction around the branch of the V at the left side of the chest.

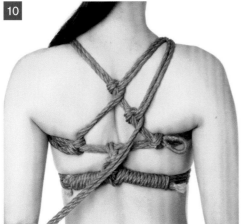

10 Return to the back side over the right shoulder, and form a cross friction.

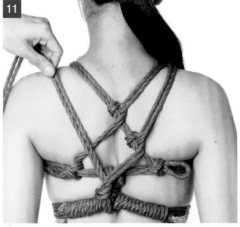

11 Hook the rope around the middle point in the back.

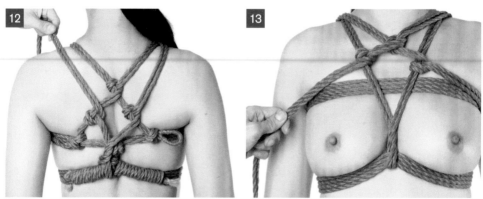

12 Pull the working section towards the Rope Bottom's left shoulder, and form a cross friction.

13 Pull the rope over the left shoulder, then form two more cross frictions.

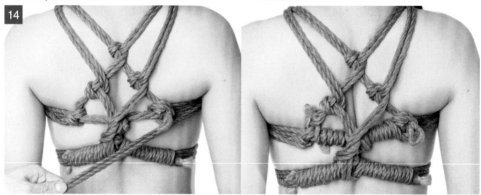

14 Pass the rope under the right armpit towards the back, and affix it in the middle. Wrap the leftover rope around the rope ring. Tuck the rope head into a gap between ropes.

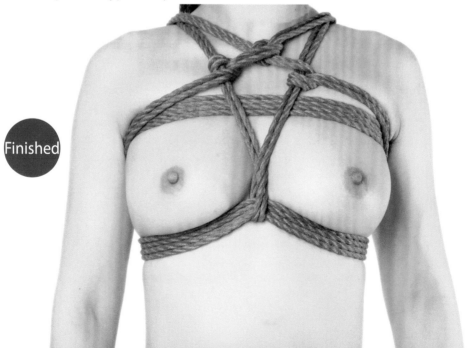

Finished

6.4 Futomomo (Thigh) Tie

Futomomo literally translates as thigh. The futomomo tie bends the leg, binding the thigh and calf together. It can be readily used in many situations. Simple futomomo ties use the double column tie from section 4.2. This section introduces another, more secure method that I often use.

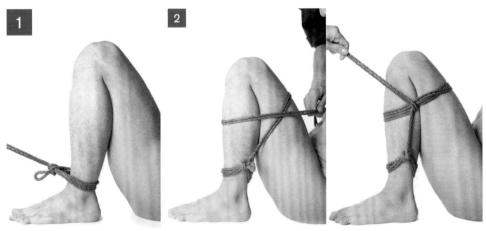

1 Form a single column tie around the ankle.

2 From outside to inside, wrap the rope twice around the thigh. Then, from inside to outside, hook the rope in the middle. If the ropes twist, tidy them after step 4.

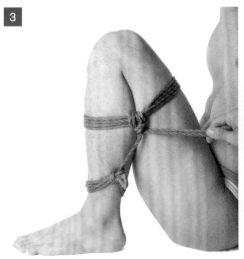

3 Form a figure 8 friction in the middle.

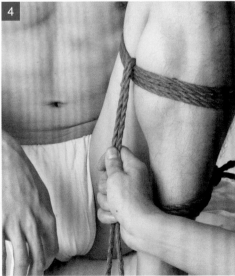

4 Pass the working end into and through the gap between the thigh and the calf, and pull through.

5

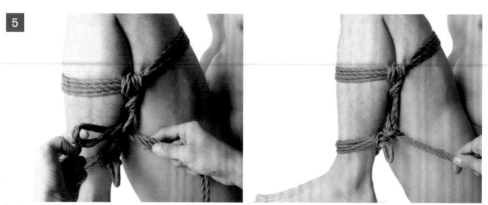

5 Return the rope to the original side, and form a twisted cross friction in the middle in order to affix the tie.

At this point, the leftover rope can be used to affix the thigh to another location. To form an extra rope ring around the thigh to make the rope bottom more comfortable, you can continue with the following steps.

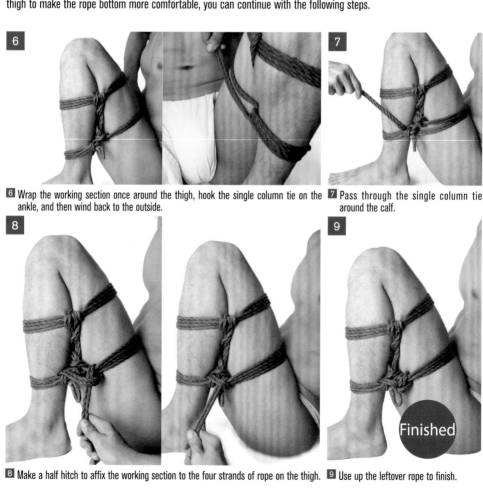

6 Wrap the working section once around the thigh, hook the single column tie on the ankle, and then wind back to the outside.

7 Pass through the single column tie around the calf.

8 Make a half hitch to affix the working section to the four strands of rope on the thigh.

9 Use up the leftover rope to finish.

6.4.1 Letter M Open-Leg Tie

Have the Rope Bottom sit on a sturdy chair, and tie both legs with the futomomo tie. Use the double half hitch method in section 4.3 to attach the futomomo to each armrest of the chair or some other immobile object, thereby forming the letter M open-leg tie.

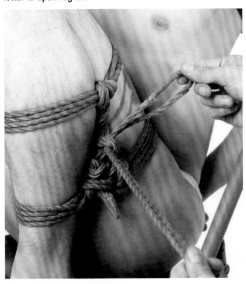 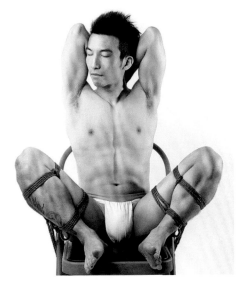

6.4.2 Crab Tie

Tie both legs with the futomomo tie, and use the leftover rope to tie each hand, thereby forming the crab tie.

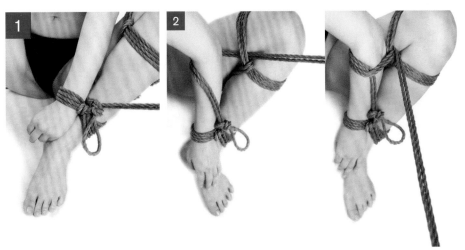

1 Use a single column tie to bind the wrist, then affix it to the rope ring around the ankle.

2 Pass the working section through the rope ring around the thigh, and then wrap twice around the forearm.

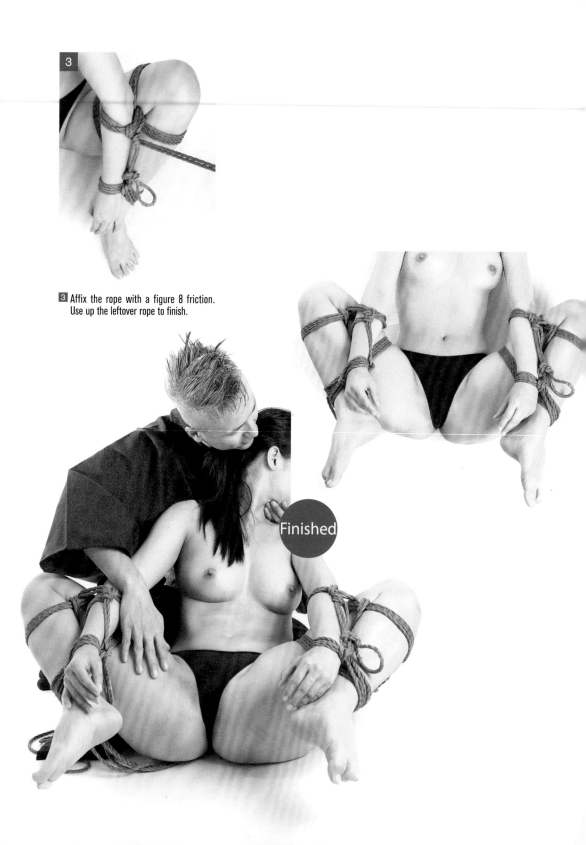

3 Affix the rope with a figure 8 friction.
Use up the leftover rope to finish.

Finished

6.5 Tortoise Shell Tie/Rhombus Rope

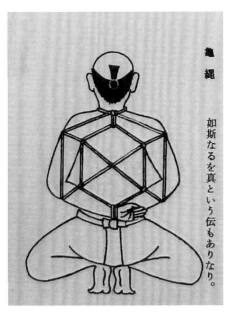

如斯なるを真という伝もありなり。

亀縄

"Kamenawa" of the Taisho-ryu school of Hojojutsu.

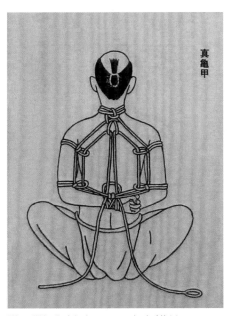

真亀甲

"Mana Kikkou" of the Ittatsu-ryu school of Hojojutsu.

Tortoise shell tie/rhombus tie is unlike other kinbaku. This may be because it can be secretly worn under ordinary clothing, or because it is often the first image that people think of when the general public thinks of Japanese SM. It has a beautiful appearance, with its ornamental nature often exceeding its restraining function. Its method of construction is also different than other techniques in this book. There are many variations out there, including some that can be tied by rope bottoms themselves. This section shows one such technique.

The term "kikkou" is often used to describe a hexagonal ornamentation in hojojutsu: for example, "kikkou musubi" [tortoise shell tie] in Ogasawara-ryu school, and "mana kikkou" [true tortoise shell] in Ittatsu-ryu school. These techniques are quite different from the "tortoise shell tie" in present-day usage. Many people wonder why the rhombus-shaped embellishment in this body harness is also called "tortoise shell tie." Master K, the author of *The Beauty of Kinbaku*, thinks that since the "kamenawa" [tortoise rope] of the Taisho-ryu school of hojojutsu includes the rhombus shape, the name has been borrowed to refer to the "tortoise shell tie" of the present day. Some people advocate that ties that only have rhombus-shaped embellishment should be called "rhombus rope," while ties that have actual hexagonal shapes should be called tortoise shell ties. However, I do not think it is necessary to differentiate these terms. I encourage readers to improvise their ties, rather than worry about the terms.

For the Rope Bottom shown here, we used more than 10 meters (33 feet) of rope to form the tortoise shell tie. The 8 meter (26 foot) rope that we often use has just the minimum length for this tie. These instructions demonstrate a method that uses two pieces of 8 meter (26 foot) rope. If you have longer rope available, then you don't need to connect ropes.

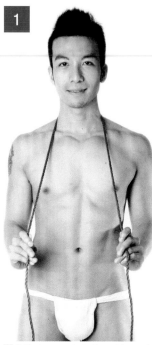

1 Fold the rope in half, and hang the midpoint around the back of the neck.

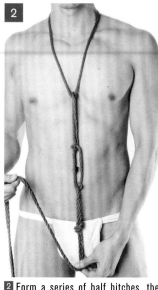

2 Form a series of half hitches, the number and position of each based on the person's body. Usually, the first knot is placed around the middle of the chest. Some people enjoy placing knots near the genitals for stimulation.

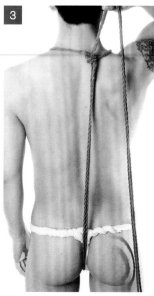

3 Pass the rope through the crotch, bring it up, hook the rope head at the back of the neck, then either tie it, or form a cross friction to hold tension. Do not make the rope too tight; you need to leave room for the rhombus shapes.

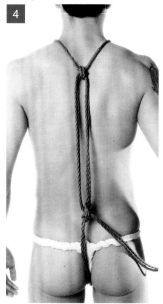

4 If you are using an 8 meter (26 foot) rope, then affix the rope at the waist with a double half hitch, to be used again later. Otherwise, you can go directly to step 6.

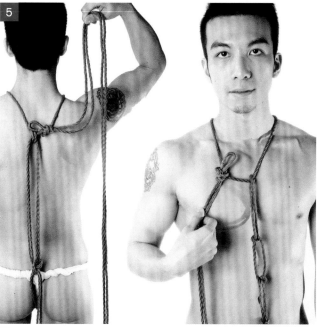

5 Start again with another piece of rope, and use the rope head to form a knot at the back of the neck. When engaging in self-bondage, one can form the knot at the front, and then slide the rope to the back.

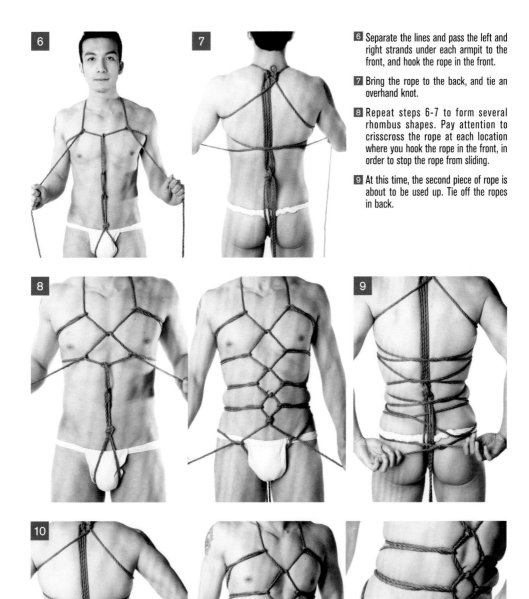

6 Separate the lines and pass the left and right strands under each armpit to the front, and hook the rope in the front.

7 Bring the rope to the back, and tie an overhand knot.

8 Repeat steps 6-7 to form several rhombus shapes. Pay attention to crisscross the rope at each location where you hook the rope in the front, in order to stop the rope from sliding.

9 At this time, the second piece of rope is about to be used up. Tie off the ropes in back.

10 Begin to use the leftover rope from step 4. One possible way is to wrap around the thigh, forming a cross friction on the outside of the thigh.

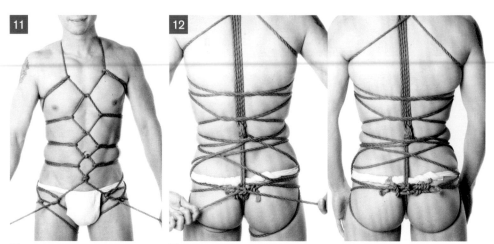

11 Use the leftover rope to decorate, until you have about 40 cm (16 inches) left for each strand.

12 Form a knot in the back, wrapping around other lines to finish.

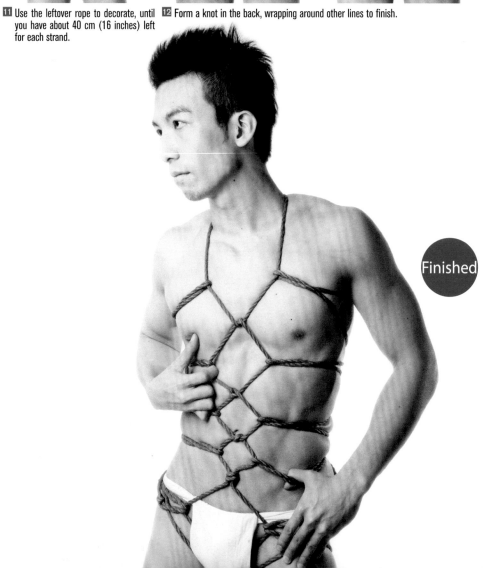

Finished

6.6 Arm Binder Tie

The October 1954 issue of the Kitan Club magazine published three photographs showing a model in an arm binder tie. The author Tsujimura Takashi named the tie "henkei ushirode shibari" [variant hands behind the back tie], and noted that it was inspired by a hands behind the back tie modeled by a pony slave in an American magazine. What he may have seen is possibly the work of the famous American bondage artist, John Willie. Generally speaking, this style of tie is regarded as one that has a special American flavor.

When both hands are held straight together behind the back, not only are the arms pressured, but the axillary brachial plexus (armpit nerve bundle) is also compressed. This is a tie that can easily cause aching and numbing, making it difficult to maintain for a prolonged period of time. The rope Top needs to pay more attention to the rope bottom's reactions. Avoid wrapping ropes around joints, and tie areas with thick musculature. If the rope bottom shows symptoms of nerve compression, immediately adjust the rope ring's position, or release the them from the bondage.

1. Have the Rope Bottom place both hands behind their back and hold them together, and tie the wrists with a double column tie.

2. Wrap the rope once around the forearms. To prevent the rope from sliding off, wrap a second time, on top of the previous wrap.

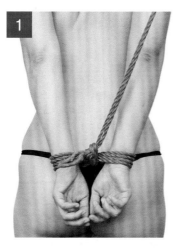

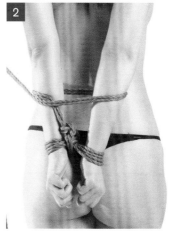

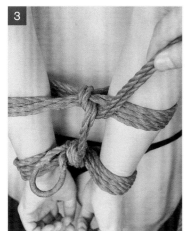

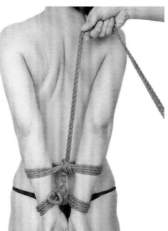

3. Adjust the rope to make it into a flat and tidy surface, and slide the crossing point in step 2 to the middle of the backside. Lastly use Figure 8 friction to hold all eight strands of rope in place.

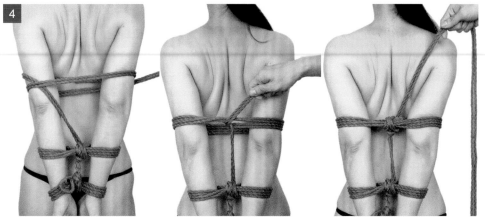

4 Using the same technique, form a rope ring around the upper arm. Use the same type of Figure 8 friction to hold all strands of rope in place.

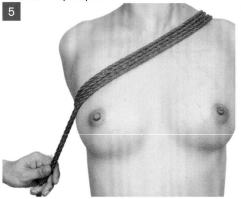

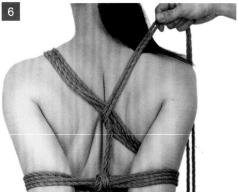

5 Pass the rope over the Rope Bottom's left shoulder, then pass the rope under the right armpit and wind to the backside. Wrap a second time to form a rope ring.

6 From the inside to the outside, hook the middle rope. Pull the rope through with your non-dominant hand, using the dominant hand to lay the ropes flat and tidy.

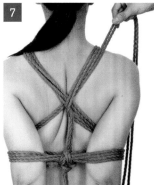

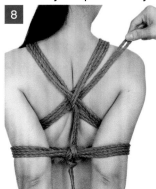

7 Pass the rope over the Rope Bottom's right shoulder, and then pass it under the left armpit and wind to the backside. Wrap a second time to form a rope ring. Weave at the front side as you go to create the figure shown.

8 Hook the rope in the middle of the backside. Pull the rope through with your non-dominant hand, using the dominant hand to adjust tension and lay the ropes flat and tidy.

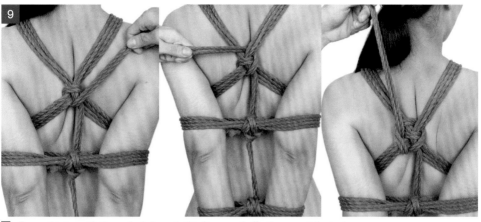

9 Form a friction with the method shown in this figure, and affix the rope at the back.

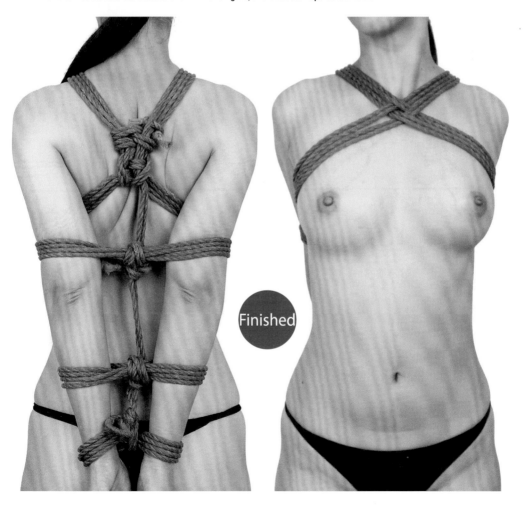

Finished

6.6.1 Strappado Tie

The posture that pulls the Rope Bottom's both arms up from behind her back is named strappado in the West. In Medieval Europe, when a prisoner was being tortured, this method was used to suspend the prisoner off the ground, pulling on the arms until the joints were dislocated. In modern BDSM, this posture is often imitated. For most rope bottoms, the arm binder tie is already prone to cause aching and numbing. The strappado posture is more demanding, so please use it with caution. Do not pull only on the Rope Bottom's hands, as shown in Figure ①. If they slip and fall, their arms can be dislocated, like in medieval times. The correct technique is to tie additional supporting rope on to the rope bottom, as in Figure ②. The slanted rope rings around the shoulders in this section are designed for this function. You can also adopt other forms of chest ties to accomplish the same thing.

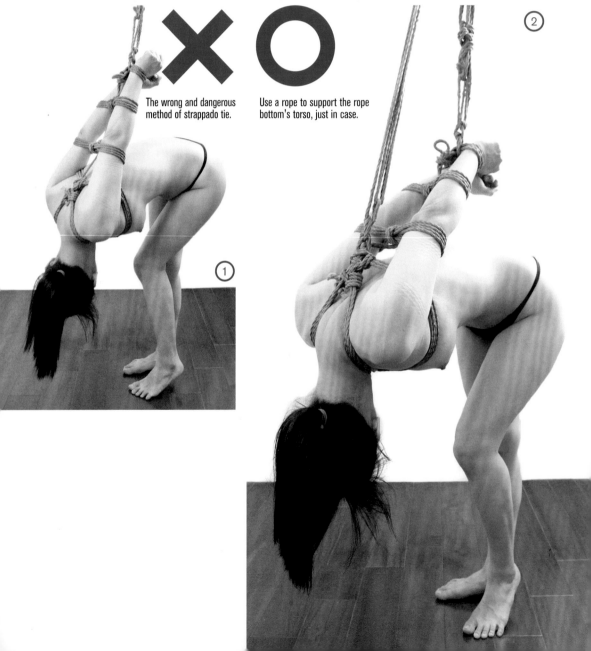

The wrong and dangerous method of strappado tie.

Use a rope to support the rope bottom's torso, just in case.

6.7 Shoulder Carrying Pole Carrier Tie

Long bamboo poles or wooden poles are very handy for bondage. The abbreviated name for tying the rope bottom to a club or cudgel is "bou shibari" [club tie]. Some people call the technique of this section "tenbinbou kazuki shibari" [shoulder carrying pole carrier tie]. The main difficulty of incorporating a pole to the tie is preventing the knots from sliding while also making sure not to tie too tight. This technique attempts to use multiple wraps to increate friction.

1 Form a single column tie around the wrist.

2 Form a cross friction around the bamboo pole.

3 Wrap the rope an extra time as shown in this figure, pulling the rope tight to affix it in place.

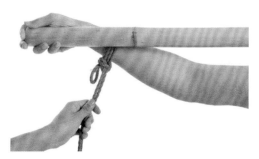

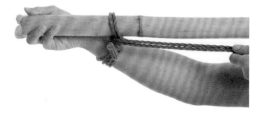

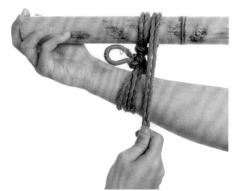

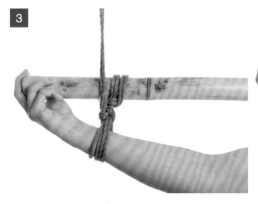

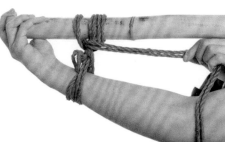

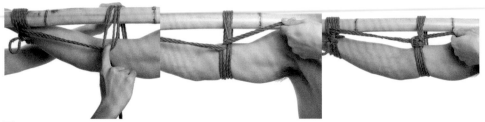

4 Form a rope ring around the arm and the bamboo pole, and affix the rope in place with a figure 8 friction. This rope ring is only used to hold the arm in place, and should not grasp the arm too tightly.

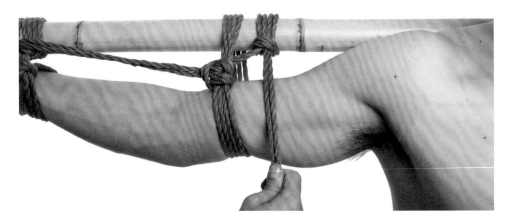

Finished

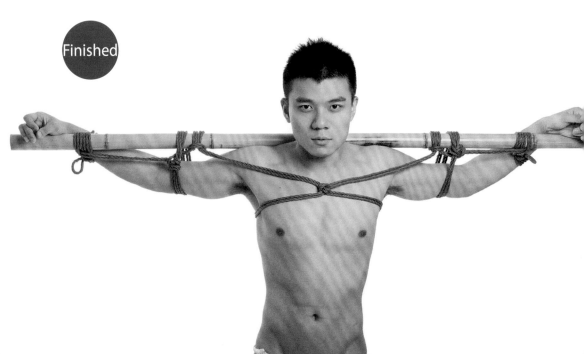

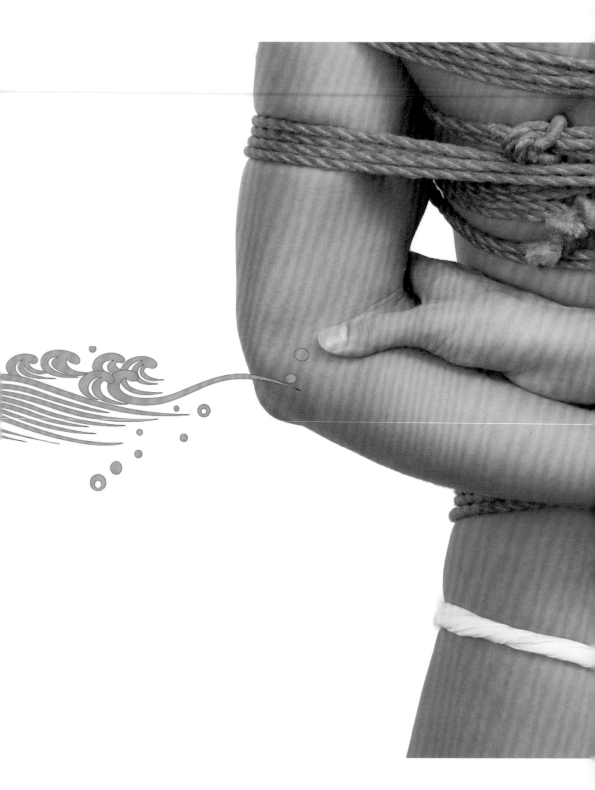

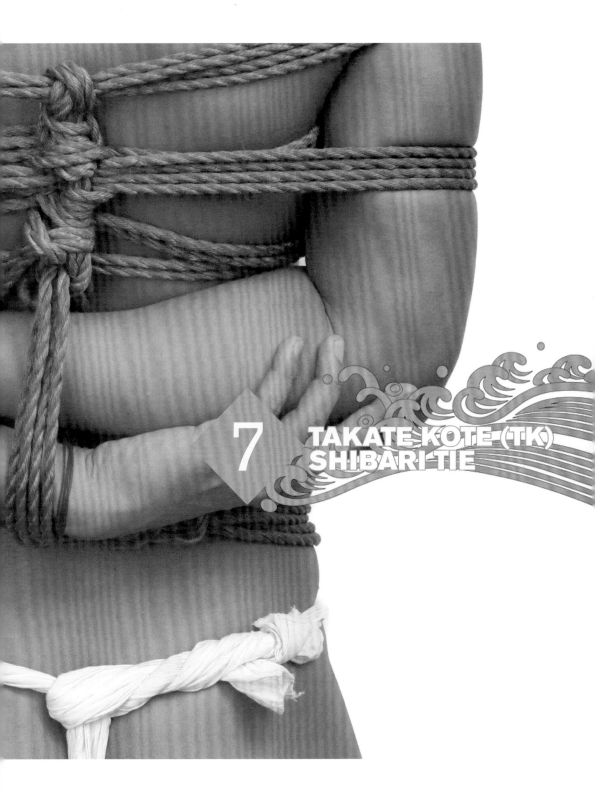

7 TAKATE KOTE (TK) SHIBARI TIE

"Takate kote shibari" is a collective name for a number of ties. This style of technique is considered the core of modern Japanese bondage, and also serves as a touchstone for the skill level of a bondage practitioner. Other names for this tie include "ushirode shibari" [hands behind the back tie] and "ushirode takete kote shibari" [hands behind the back, forearms and upper arms tie], amongst others. Some people think the nomenclature is due to the rope bottom's hands being fixed to the back (ushirode: hands behind the back), with the tying of both the forearms (kote: forearms) and the upper arms (takate: upper arms). However, there are other people that think "takate" means pulling the forearms high. These people tend to call the tie in this section ushirode shibari, while believing that in takate kote shibari the forearms should be pulled up to a higher position than what is shown in this section.

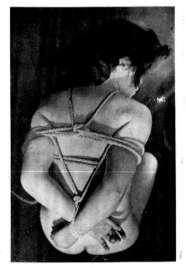

こんな繩の掛け方は如何
ですか、いささか繩が多過
ぎるきらいはありますが、
首へかけた繩で両方の二の
腕を締めつけ、更に両手首
へ通蓋させたもので、胸に
は散意に全然繩を刺さな
った。これは両胸がぐっと
せばめられて後の鯵輪
いるので後手の中でも鯵縛
感が特に強くあらわれてい
るものの一つであると思う

"Ushirode to Takate Kote ni yoru Kinbakubi no Kousatsu" [A Study of the Beauty of Bondage by Means of Hands Behind the Back and Takate-Kote] by Tsujimura Takashi and Tsukamoto Tetsuzou. April 1953 issue of Kitan Club. The bondage pattern at the backside still has a strong hojojutsu style.

At any rate, takate kote shibari appears to be the most common Japanese name for this tie. In the English language circle, since both the Rope Bottom's arms are held together at right angles, this tie used to be called "box tie." Recently the name has been borrowed from the Japanese phonetics takate-kote, and then simplified as "TK." Generally speaking, TK needs about two pieces of rope, so some people call this tie "2TK." In the next section, we will introduce a "3TK" tie that uses three pieces of rope. This kind of naming convention may not make sense entirely, but it appears that the name has been customarily established by popular usage.

Tracing the source of this tie, it is found that in Japanese hojojutsu, a common technique is to tie a prisoner's wrists and forearms, and affix both hands of the prisoner to their back. However, takate kote shibari does not appear to be the formal name of a tie from any hojojutsu school or style. It is likely a casual name from the Edo period.

Having been revised by nawashi in modern times, the takate kote shibari of contemporary kinbaku is very different from traditional hojojutsu. Its primary characteristics include: hands tied behind the back, forearms placed parallel, and elbows bent at ninety degrees. It uses rope folded in half to form on the upper torso at least two large rope rings that are approximately parallel, with each rope ring being formed by wrapping the rope twice or more.

For its design, takate kote shibari attempts to satisfy two principles that run counter to each other: on the one hand the tie needs to preserve the appearance of the traditional hojojutsu; on the other hand the tie also needs to avoid bringing too much suffering to the Rope Bottom during suspension. Traditional hojojutsu was designed to prevent prisoners from escaping, and is bound to make the Rope Bottom uncomfortable. Therefore, takate kote shibari tries to achieve, as much as possible, a balance between a number of variables. Each step and detail has a practical rationale behind it.

Takate kote shibari is the first major obstacle that a student of kinbaku will encounter. A beginner may manage to memorize the sequential steps of this tie in a short amount of time, and produce a tie that has a similar appearance to the real thing. However, if you want to do suspension, then you need to practice over and over to grasp the finer details of the technique. Many people think the learning the takate kote shibari needs to be guided in a one-on-one, face-to-face fashion, in order to achieve a comprehensively complete result for everyone's safety.

Contemporary investigation has led to many people pointing out that takate kote shibari is not necessarily the best way to do suspension bondage with regards to human body mechanics. However, due to its historical status and representative nature, this tie has become the most important component of Japanese bondage aesthetics. Without takate kote shibari, the tie will lack its Japanese flavor!

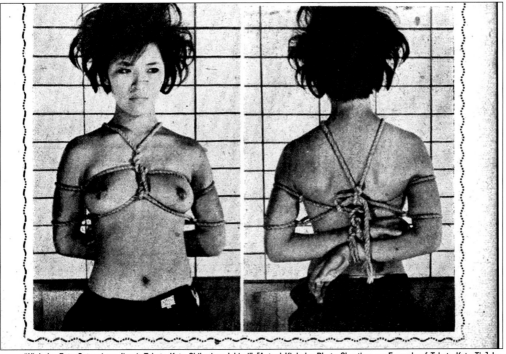

"Kinbaku Foto Satsuei no Jissai: Takate Kote Shibari no Ichirei" [Actual Kinbaku Photo Shooting: an Example of Takate Kote Tie] by Tsukamoto Tetsuzou. September 1961 issue of Kitan Club. This tie already has the appearance that is similar to the modern takate kote tie, but the bondage under the armpits is not kannuki, and instead is the half hitch to lock the arms tight. This is probably also a vestige from hojojutsu.

7.1 Basic Form

Most schools of kinbaku have their own technique for takate kote shibari. The technique demonstrated in this book is done by people such as Akechi Denki and Kanna, and has been quite popular around the world in recent years. This section will introduce the basic form of the tie, and the next section will introduce additional embellishment and decoration.

7.1.1 Steps of the Tie

1 The purpose of steps 1-7 is to form a single column tie on both of the Rope Bottom's forearms. Have the rope bottom place both hands behind his back, with forearms parallel while relaxing their shoulders. He should extend both palms to the opposite sides of his body as much as possible without straining himself.

2 Pass the rope head upward to pass through the space between the Rope Bottom's arms and torso, and pull the rope head to the height of the neck.

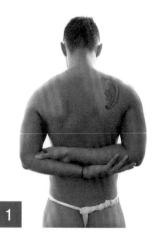
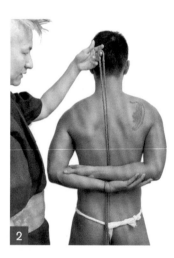

3 Wrap the rope once around the arms.

4 Let the rope head end drop down, and fold the working section (that has been pulled upward) back on itself, holding the rope with the non-dominant hand as shown in the image. Pay attention to the position of the thumb and the rope tail section.

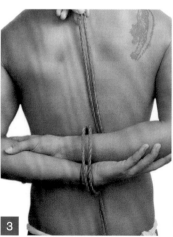
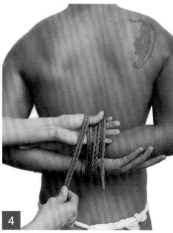

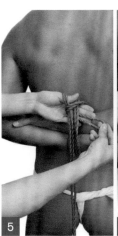

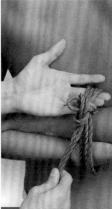

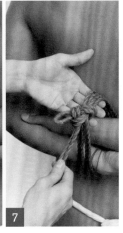

5 Cross the rope head over all of the ropes, then pass it under all of the ropes. A loop will form around the thumb of the non-dominant hand.

6 Pass the rope head through the loop.

7 Pull tight.

British nawashi Wykd Dave uses this tie, which is also referred to as a "fast bowline." Its merit is the simple and fast hand movement, but the rope tail may still be pulled straight under strong tension. This tie is sufficient for the forearms in takate kote shibari.

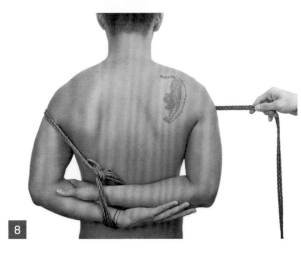

By placing the forearms parallel with wrists facing each other, the goal is to prevent compressing the nerves of the wrists. The single column tie on the forearms should leave a gap that is at least two fingers wide to allow enough space for the Rope Bottom to exchange hand positions.

There are 3 goals in step 10: Ⓐ adjust the rope ring to an ideal level; Ⓑ adjust the rope ring to make it flat and neat; Ⓒ adjust the crossing position to hook in the middle. This can be very difficult. Beginners, and some experienced rope Tops, may need to adjust this step many times. Some nawashi adjust the crossing position after finishing step 11, and others do not.

8 Wrap the rope over the Rope Bottom's upper arm. In the example here, the rope is wrapped clockwise over the rope bottom's left arm.

9 Wind the second wrap below the first wrap, and let the rope cross on the rope bottom's left shoulder.

10 Stand behind the Rope Bottom, and use your dominant hand to hook the rope from the inside to the outside. With your non-dominant hand, insert your index and middle fingers into the rope ring to adjust for even tension and help the ropes lay flat. Finally, pull the rope to center the friction over the Rope Bottom's spine.

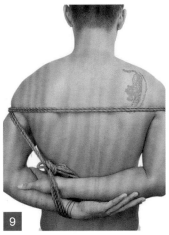

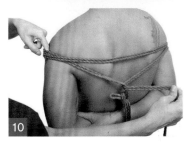

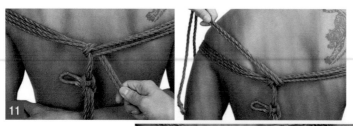
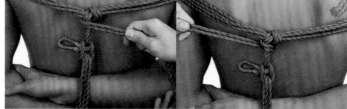

11 Affix the rope with a figure 8 friction. This part of rope is called the "stem," and this first rope ring is the "upper wrap."

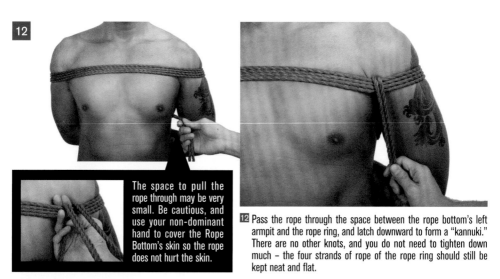

The space to pull the rope through may be very small. Be cautious, and use your non-dominant hand to cover the Rope Bottom's skin so the rope does not hurt the skin.

12 Pass the rope through the space between the rope bottom's left armpit and the rope ring, and latch downward to form a "kannuki." There are no other knots, and you do not need to tighten down much – the four strands of rope of the rope ring should still be kept neat and flat.

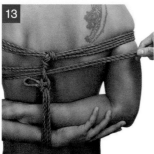
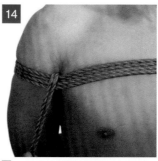
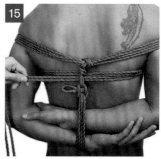

13 Bring the rope to the back, and pass under the stem.

14 Pass the rope between the Rope Bottom's right armpit and the rope ring, and cinch downward to form a kannuki.

15 Bring the rope to the back, and pass through under the stem.

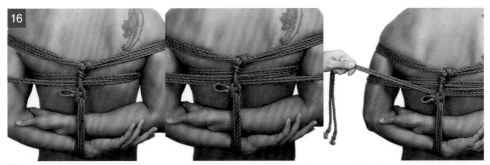

16 Wrap the rope around the Rope Bottom's arms twice to form a second rope ring. Pay attention that the rope should pass under the stem. These wraps will form the second rope ring, called the "lower wrap."

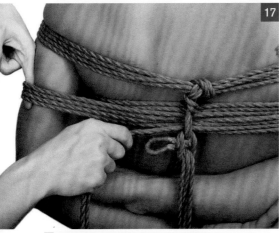

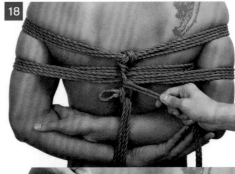

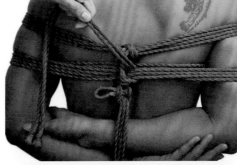

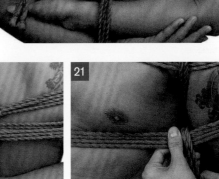

17 Stand behind the rope bottom, and use your dominant hand to hook the rope from the inside to the outside. With your non-dominant hand, insert your index and middle fingers into the rope ring to even tension and help the ropes lay flat. This tension should be the same as the upper wrap.

18 In steps 18-20, we will attach the lower wrap to the stem. First, cross the rope head over the stem, and hook upwards from the bottom under the four strands of the lower wrap. Pay attention not to hook the horizontal ropes from step 11.

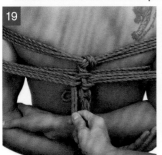

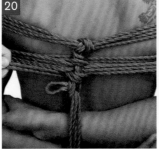

19 Cross the rope head end over the stem, and hook downwards the four strands of rope of the lower wrap.

20 Wrap once, from the outside to the inside around the stem, and pull towards the left.

21 Pass the rope between the Rope Bottom's left arm and body, and cinch downward to form a kannuki.

TAKATE KOTE (TK) SHIBARI TIE — **BASIC FORM** — **7**

22 Bring the rope to the back, and pass under the stem.

23 Pass the rope through the space between the rope bottom's right arm and body, and cinch downward to form a kannuki.

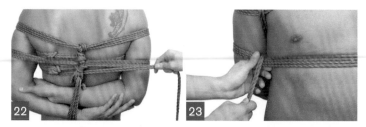

24 Bring the rope to the back, and affix the rope on the stem with knot. Use up the leftover rope by wrapping.

This section shows that the Rope Top's dominant hand is his right hand, and wraps are done clockwise. For left-handed rope Tops, consider wrapping counterclockwise. This is not universal – there are renowned nawashi who are right-handed but wrap counter-clockwise. Most people feel this is personal preference, and neither way is better than the other.

Finished

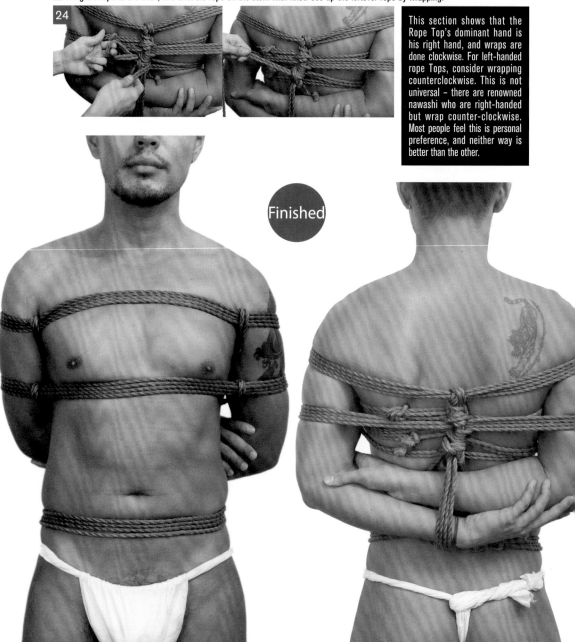

7.1.2 **Finer Points**

The basic structure of takate kote shibari is centered on the stem. To attach the rope bottom's upper body to some fixture, we often use another piece of rope to tie an overhand knot on the stem (see Figure ①), or for further safety, tie a Carrick bend around the stem. When performing suspension, we often suspend the stem, wherein the upper wrap and the lower wrap can tightly grip the upper body (see Figure ②). The corresponding basic kinbaku principle should be this: for each of the upper wrap and the lower wrap, the four strands of rope need to be aligned into a flat surface, and the rope tension should remain uniform. Also, the rope tension of the upper wraps should be the same as that of the lower wraps. The purpose of the figure 8 friction in step 11 and the "half-moon friction" in steps 18-20 is to firmly grab the four rope strands of the upper and lower wraps into a bundle.

The kannuki in steps 12, 14, 21, and 23 helps ensure safety: the upper wrap kannuki prevents the wrap from sliding upwards above the shoulders and strangling the neck. However, the armpit is where the brachial plexus passes through, so a kannuki placed here may compress the nerves. The four kannuki cinches should be just enough to hook onto the rope, and should not be pulled too tight.

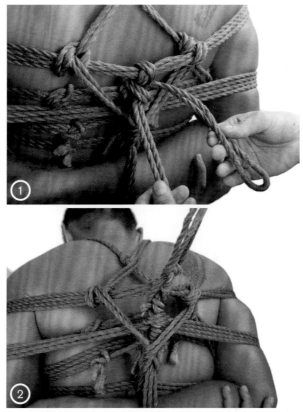

The stem should be positioned in the middle of the rope bottom's back. Only then will balance be achieved during suspension, thereby avoiding putting too much force on one side. If you are not sure where to place the stem, you can touch to locate the rope bottom's spine.

There are many other nawashi who do not form kannuki on the upper wrap at all, and opt for other ways to keep the upper wrap in place. The kannuki on the lower wrap can work to secure the rope structure, and also has the effect of compressing and pushing out the breasts. At present, most nawashi prefer to keep this lower wrap kannuki. Since there is naturally some space between the arms and the body, while forming the lower wrap kannuki, you can slightly tighten the lower wrap, but you still need to keep the four strands of rope neat and flat.

In principle, the above four kannuki cinches should not be burdened with too much body weight, in order to prevent the upper and lower wraps from being pulled too tightly. Therefore, in steps 11, 13, and 20, the rope should all be passed under the stem. As seen in Figure ②, only the two rope rings (upper and lower wraps) are pulled up along with the stem; the kannuki cinches should not be included among them. In steps 12, 14, 21, and 23, each kannuki should be cinched downward, from top to bottom. If the kannuki is cinched upward, from bottom to top, it will cause the rope to cross itself at the back or under the armpit (see Figure ③ on the next page), and increase the risk of causing discomfort.

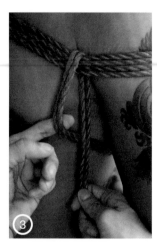
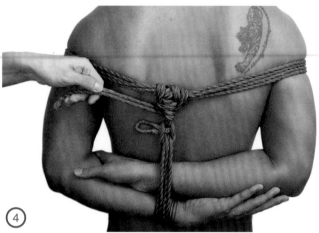

Generally speaking, the basic form of TK will use two pieces of hemp rope, with need to connect the ropes in the midst of tying. Rope connection should occur at the backside of the Rope Bottom as much as possible. First, this is for the sake of safety (preventing the knot from pressing against the body); for this reason, avoid connecting ropes on the arm, under the armpit, against the side of the body, or close to the ribs. Second, this is for aesthetics, as people do not wish to see the connection knot at the front of the body. Since everyone's body type is different, the nawashi should adapt according to circumstances. If the rope connection is about to occur at the front or the side of the body, one way to deal with this is to wrap the rope a few more times at the backside (see Figure ④), in order to use up a small section of the rope. Alternatively, you can use the square knot in Section 4.5.2 to connect the ropes.

As you finish the TK of this section, you may find that there is a lot of rope left over. As long as it does not affect the function, you can use the leftover rope for decoration. The decorating method varies according to different individuals and styles. We will introduce some examples in the next section.

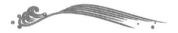

Must TK be done very quickly?
Why is speed of the essence?

When I was learning kinbaku, nawashi Kanna demand the students to finish the basic TK tie in under two minutes thirty seconds. With decoration, the tie should be finished under three minutes thirty seconds. Of course, every small detail still needs to meet the standard. Tying quickly shows a level of agility, while reducing the wait time for the audience and Rope Model. It also indicates the Rope Top has achieved a certain level of proficiency. For the sake of safety, one must at least achieve this standard of tying before even attempting suspension bondage.

Even though you may have developed an ability to tie quickly through practice and training, it does not mean you have to tie quickly. If you aim is to enjoy the delightfulness of kinbaku, it would be better to tie slowly, as in shown in Chapter 3 "Delightful Kinbaku." The nawashi Pedro Diniz Reis once said, "Some people spend five minutes to have sex, while others enjoy lovemaking for an hour." Even on stage, a nice performance also needs varying speeds and rhythms, using slow speed to express emotions, and fast rhythm to convey power. It is only with such variations that one may grab the audience's attention. As always, safety always overrides speed.

7.1.3 Prevention of Nerve Compression

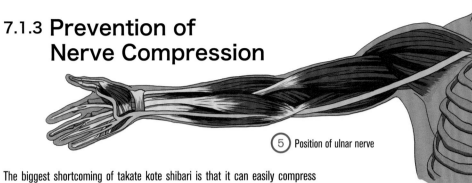

(5) Position of ulnar nerve

The biggest shortcoming of takate kote shibari is that it can easily compress the nerves in the arms. Rope bondage practitioners in the West have done a lot of research on this topic, in order to reduce suffering, and lower the risk of injuries. This section shares some result of their research.

The brachial plexus extends from the torso towards the arm, and splits into three branches. Running relatively deep, the median nerve is rarely affected by rope bondage. The ulnar nerve and the radial nerve are what we should devote more attention to.

Extending from the shoulder, the ulnar nerve follows along the bottom side of the arm until it reaches the tip of the little finger (see Figure ⑤). The ulnar nerve can be affected by the single column tie on the forearms. We advise Rope Bottoms to raise their forearms slightly, so that the two forearms remain parallel. Some people feel that it is more comfortable to let their arms drop (see Figure ⑥). However, over time, and especially during suspension, this scissors-like position may compress the ulnar nerves without the rope bottom noticing. The symptom is a numbing feeling of the ring fingers and the little fingers. At such a time, you can have the Rope Bottom switch positions of their hands (see Figure ⑦). Consequently, if you plan on performing suspension, this rope ring must be loose. With this degree of looseness, the rope bottom may be able to get out of the tie by herself. This shows that modern SM rope bondage is a sexual game played with informed consent. Its goal is to let the rope bottom stay comfortable, thereby prolonging the time of playing or performing. This is very different from the goal hojojutsu, which is to prevent the bound prisoner from escaping.

(6)

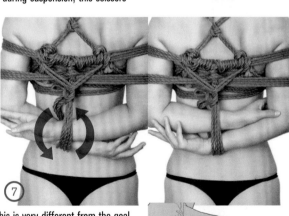

(7)

The radial nerve extends from the armpit towards the arm, and winds around the top of the triceps to the outer side of the upper arm (see Figure ⑧). With both the upper wrap and the lower wrap, it is very difficult to avoid the radial nerve completely. We can only choose some relatively safe parts to tie. The optimal position to place these wraps is a much debated topic. Rope enthusiasts in the West have conducted extensive research on this subject, but in Japan, every nawashi ties the wraps around different parts of the arms, which can puzzle Westerners.

(8) The position of radial nerve

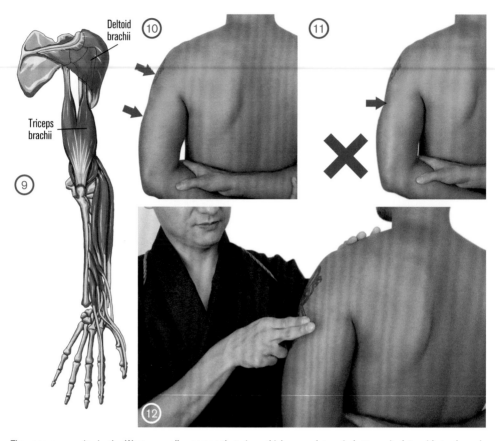

The rope community in the West generally reasons that since thick musculature is better suited to withstand rope's tension, the upper wrap can be pressed against the deltoid, while the lower wrap should be pressed against the triceps (see Figures 8 and 9). One should avoid placing the wrap between the deltoid and the triceps, in the sunken area where the musculature is relatively thin (see Figure ⑩). However, some Japanese nawashi hold the opposite view, and think that the upper wrap should be placed exactly in this sunken area in order to prevent the rope ring from slipping off. Personally, I feel the Western view makes more sense.

These are rough, general principles. Every person's nerves and blood vessels are located in different positions, just like everyone has different outward appearances and features. There is even more diversity with regard to thickness of fat tissue and strength of musculature. The safest approach may be to ask the rope bottom to place her arms into the TK position, then have the nawashi use two fingers to probe their arm from top to bottom, looking for the most sensitive, sore, or painful point (see Figure ⑫). If upon touching this point, the Rope Bottom feels like a small hammer is hitting the nerve, this area that should be avoided during bondage.

When performing rope bondage on the floor, as long as you avoid pulling the chest wraps too tight, there will be relatively little danger. Consequently, we can relax the standard of precision of where to place the chest wraps. However, during suspension, the person's body is pulled off the ground, so the parts of the body being tied will sustain tremendous tension. At such times, chest wraps cannot be too tight, in order to avoid discomfort. On the other hand, the wraps should not be too loose, either, in order to prevent the rope from sliding off. This is a test of the nawashi, and makes us appreciate performance, as well as the differences between "delightful kinbaku" and "performance kinbaku."

7.2 Decorations

After finishing the basic form of TK, the leftover rope is often used for decorations. These kinds of decorations can accentuate the curve of the body, function as a symbol of the nawashi's personal style, or reinforce the structure of the tie.

In traditional hojojutsu, in order to prevent the prisoners from learning the tie, complex ties are mostly positioned at the back of the Rope Bottom. In modern kinbaku, there are many decorative ties at the front of the body, in order to make the bondage more beautiful.

7.2.1 V Neck

This type of decoration has the effect of squeezing out the breasts, and is one of the most common decorations. The diamond-shaped decoration at the backside is often used in Akechi-ryu (Akechi Denki style).

1 Proceed to step 21 of the TK basic form. Do not tie off. Instead, form a twisted cross friction to attach the rope to the upper wrap in the vicinity of the right shoulder blade.

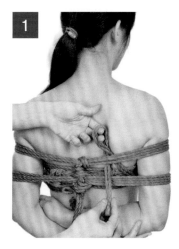
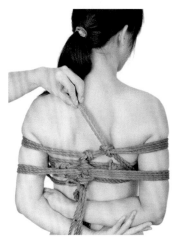

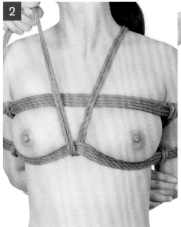
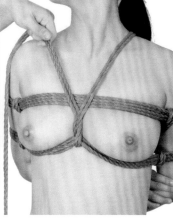

2 Pass the rope over the rope bottom's left shoulder, hook around the lower wrap between the breasts, and pull up the rope slightly. The desire here is to lift up the breasts without hurting the shoulder. Cross the rope over itself once to affix it in place.

TAKATE KOTE (TK) SHIBARI TIE   **7**   DECORATIONS

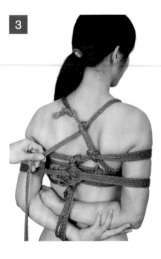

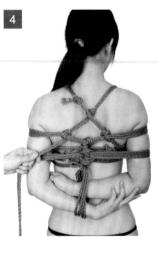

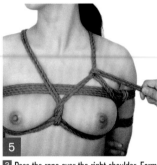

3 Pass the rope over the right shoulder. Form a cross friction with the rope from step 2.

4 Form a cross friction or twisted cross friction with the upper wrap.

5 Pass the rope under the lower wrap, and return to the front. Hook the vertical rope near the left collar bone to form a V.

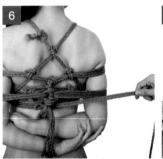

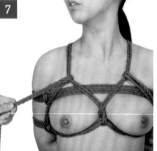

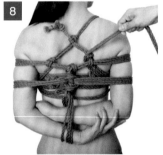

6 Bring the rope to the backside, and pass it through under the stem.

7 Pass the working end through under the lower wrap, and return it to the front. Hook the vertical strand near the left collar bone to form a V neck at the other side.

8 Follow the rope back where it came from to the backside. Wrap once around the twisted cross friction formed in step 1.

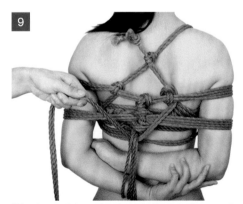

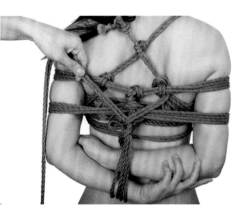

9 Hook around the single column tie above the forearms. Cross once around the rope, and adjust its position to the center.

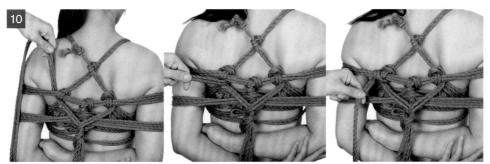

10 Wrap around the knot formed in step 4 (either cross friction or twisted cross friction).

11 Wrap to finish the leftover rope.

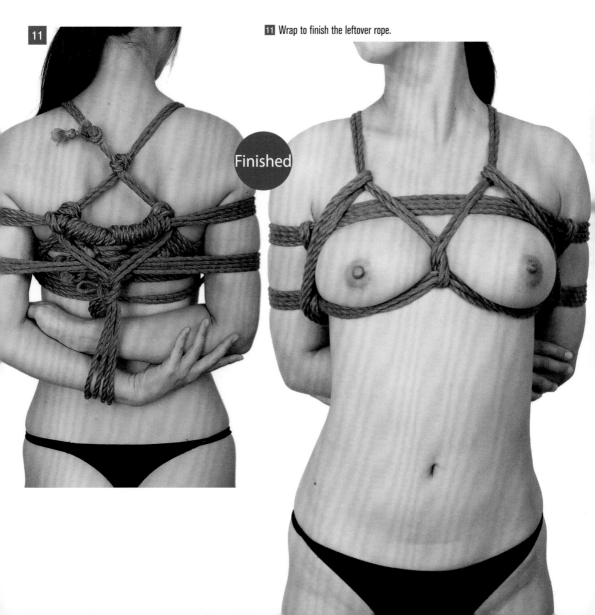

Finished

7.2.2 Akechi Denki Style –Ushoro Takete Tasuki-Gake

"Ushoro takete tasuki-gake" was designed by Akechi Denki. Tasuki is a cord that is used to tuck up the sleeves of a kimono. This TK tie gets its name from the two shoulder strands that look like tasuki. Many of Akechi Denki's ties have drawn from traditional hojojutsu and paid much attention to the aesthetics of the backside. The backside diamond-shaped decoration of this tie is a common symbol in his ties.

After the passing of Akechi Denki, this tie was at one time exclusively used by the students of Akechi-ryu, including Kanna. Later, Hajime Kinoko learned this tie from Kanna, and introduced it to Europe, where it became popular. The tie has gradually come to be seen as the "standard" TK decoration. In fact, Akechi Denki himself often changed his ties such that they evolved over time. He always reviewed his previous ties to improve his subsequent ties, and every time he performed kinbaku, his tie was different. Adhering rigidly to a fixed pattern will deviate from his spirit.

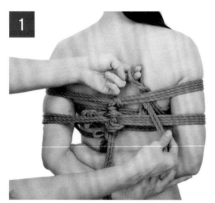
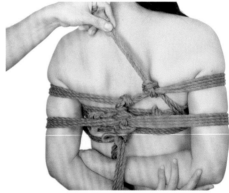

1 Proceed to step 21 of the TK basic form. Do not attach the rope to the stem. Instead, form a twisted cross friction to attach the rope to the upper wrap in the vicinity of the right shoulder blade.

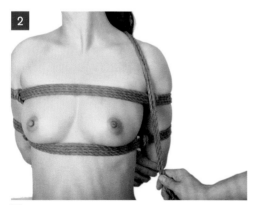
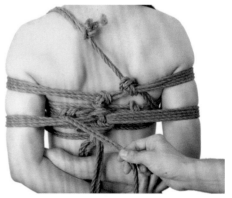

2 Pass the rope to cross over the Rope Bottom's left shoulder. Pass the rope under the lower wrap at the left side, and then through the gap above the arm to come to the backside.

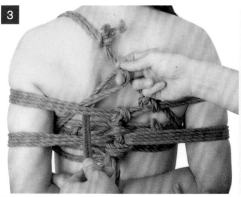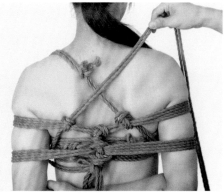

3 Bring the rope up to the vicinity of the rope bottom's left shoulder blade, and make a twisted cross knot on the upper wrap.

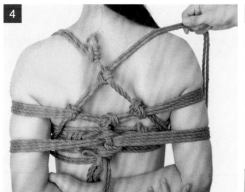

4 Cross the rope to the slanted strand of rope formed in step 1, and make a cross friction.

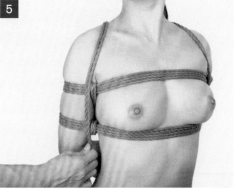

5 Cross over the right shoulder and bring the rope to the right front side. Pass the rope under the lower wrap at its right side, and then through the gap above the arm to go to the backside.

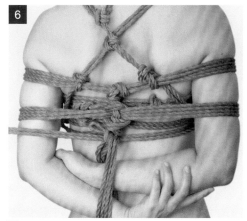

6 Pass the rope under the stem, over to the left side of the Rope Bottom.

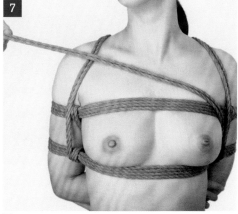

7 Pass the rope under the lower wrap at its left side, and then through the gap above the forearm, bringing the rope to the front side.

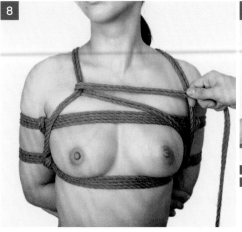

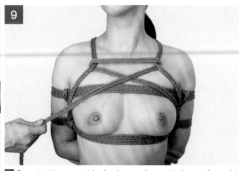

8 From inside to outside, hook onto the vertical rope formed in
9 step 5, and then go towards the left side of the Rope Bottom.

For left-right symmetry, hook onto the vertical rope formed in
step 2, this time from the outside to the inside, and then go
towards the right side of the Rope Bottom.

10 In the middle of the chest, at a position slightly above the upper
wrap, form a cross friction.

11 Pass the rope under the lower wrap at the right side, and then
through the gap above the arm to go to the backside.

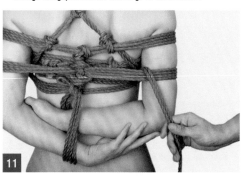

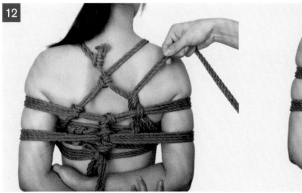
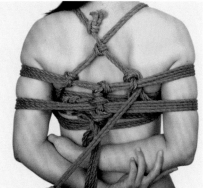

12 Wrap once around the twisted cross friction formed in step 1.

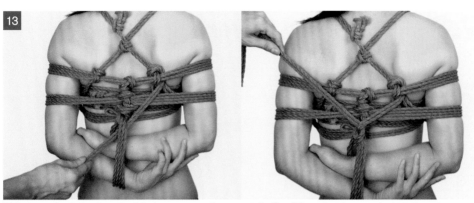

13 Hook onto the single column tie of the forearms, cross the rope onto itself, and then adjust the crossed point to the center.

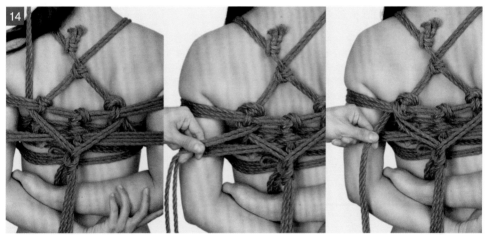

14 Wrap once around the twisted cross friction formed in step 3.

15 Wrap the leftover rope around the upper wrap, and tuck the rope tail into some gap of the upper wrap. Depending on the length of the leftover rope, you can use other techniques.

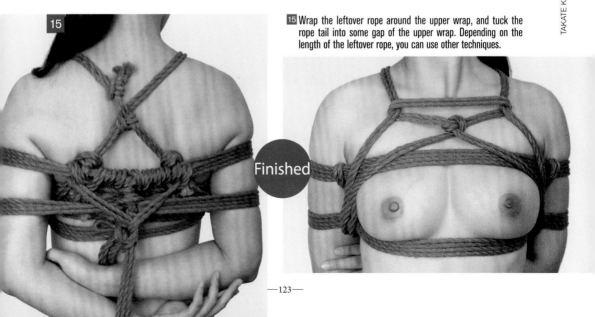

Finished

7.3 Ebi Tie and Reverse Ebi Tie

Takate kote shibari is the starting point of many common Japanese kinbaku ties. This section will demonstrate two examples.

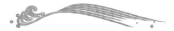

7.3.1 Agura Tie, Ebi Tie

"Ebi" means shrimp in Japanese, and "ebi-seme" [shrimp torture] is one of the torture techniques of ancient Japan. The tie forces the prisoner's body to curl forward like a shrimp, such that the upper body is pressed very closely to the feet. Most people cannot endure this posture for a long time; they will quickly become covered in sweat, in unbearable pain.

Modern Japanese kinbaku refers to this cross-legged tie as "agura shibari" [barbarian-style sitting tie] or "zazen shibari" [meditation-style sitting tie]. If both legs are tied close to the upper body, then the tie is called "ebi shibari" [shrimp tie]. The latter tie is not necessarily cross-legged, while its terminology is often used interchangeably with the agura shibari. Comparing with the ebi-seme of the ancient times, the modern ebi tie has been revised to become safer, taking on a form that does not compress the Rope B ottom that much.

This version has quite a few rope rings around the thigh and leg, in order to use the rope efficiently. In practice, you can also tie a single column tie around the lower leg first, and then immediately affix the rope at the backside. The leftover rope can be used for other purposes.

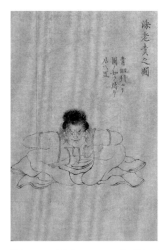

Ebi-seme (shrimp torture); Keizai Dai-hiroku [Record of Punishments]; 1850; author unknown.

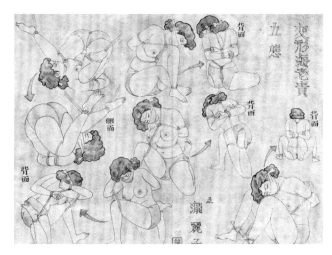

Taki Reiko, "Hen-kei Ebi-seme Go-tai" [Variations of Shrimp Torture, in Five Poses]; Kitan Club; March 1954 edition.

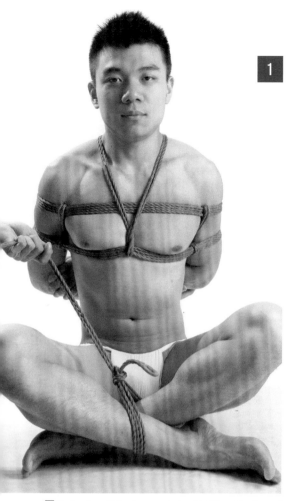

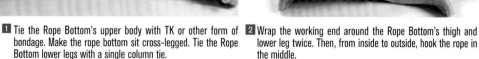

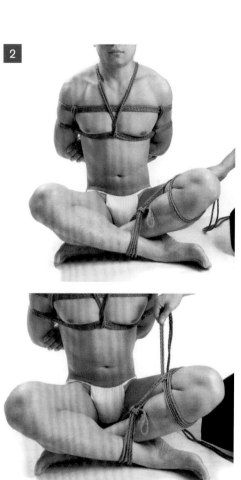

1 Tie the Rope Bottom's upper body with TK or other form of bondage. Make the rope bottom sit cross-legged. Tie the Rope Bottom lower legs with a single column tie.

2 Wrap the working end around the Rope Bottom's thigh and lower leg twice. Then, from inside to outside, hook the rope in the middle.

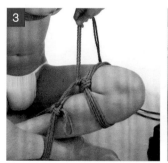

3 Affix the rope with a figure 8 friction.

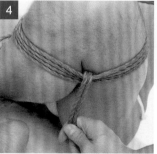

4 Pass the rope through the gap between the thigh and the lower leg, and form a kannuki.

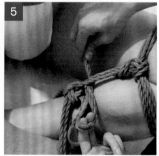

5 Pull the rope towards the middle of the body. Around the vicinity of the single column tie from step 1, form a twisted cross friction.

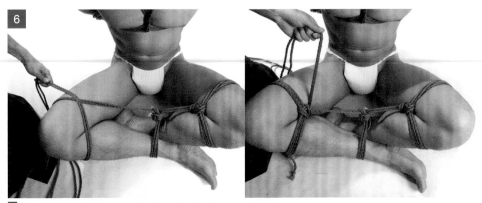

6 Around the thigh and lower leg at the other side, form the same rope ring.

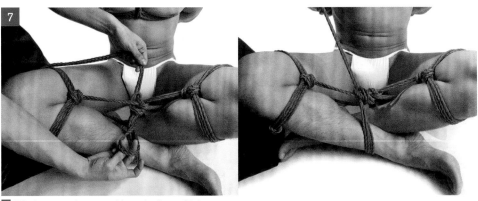

7 Affix the rope at the center with a twisted cross friction.

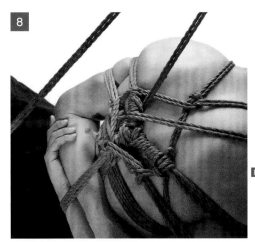

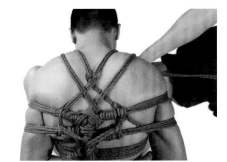

8 Cross the working end over the Rope Bottom's shoulder. Slightly force the Rope Bottom's upper body downward, and then affix the rope at the stem of the already formed TK. Notice that this step can only affix to the backside. In ancient times, the method to deal with a prisoner wrapped the rope around his neck, but doing so will hurt the Rope Bottom's cervical vertebrae.

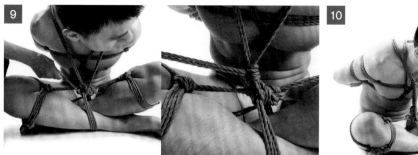

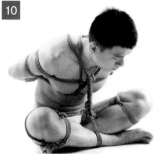

9 Hook the rope around the single column tie around the low legs, and affix it with a double half hitch.

10 Wind the leftover rope to use it up.

Finished

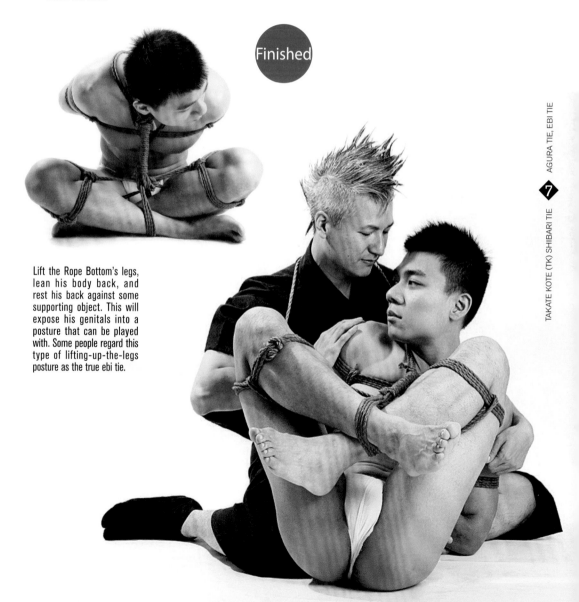

Lift the Rope Bottom's legs, lean his body back, and rest his back against some supporting object. This will expose his genitals into a posture that can be played with. Some people regard this type of lifting-up-the-legs posture as the true ebi tie.

7.3.2 Reverse Ebi Tie

Making the Rope Bottom curl backwards is called "reverse ebi tie." This is a position is often used in suspension bondage. This section demonstrates a type of reverse ebi tie that does not lift the Rope Bottom off the ground. To do so, you need different supporting ropes. At first glance, this posture looks like the "hogtie" that is often seen in Western bondage. The latter tie often ties the Rope Bottom's hands and feet at her back, rather that tying the feet to a chest harness.

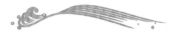

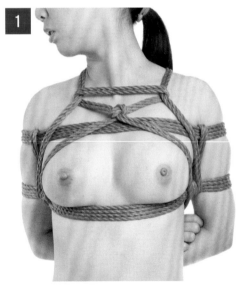

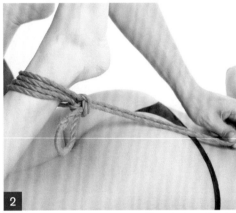

1 Tie the Rope Bottom's upper body with TK or other form of bondage.

2 Make the Rope Bottom lie face down. Form a single column tie around her lower leg.

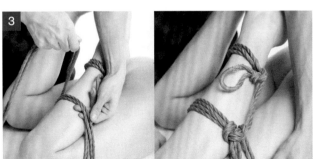

3 Form a rope ring around her thigh and lower leg, and affix the rope with a figure 8 friction.

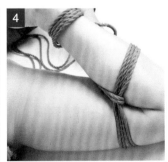

4 Form a kannuki cinch on the inside.

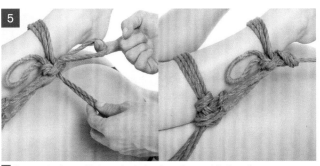
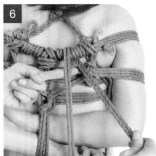

5 Form a twisted cross friction at the single column tie around the lower leg.

6 Hook the working end around the upper wrap.

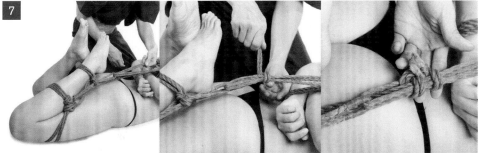

7 Hook the rope through the rope head at the lower leg, and affix the rope with a double half hitch.

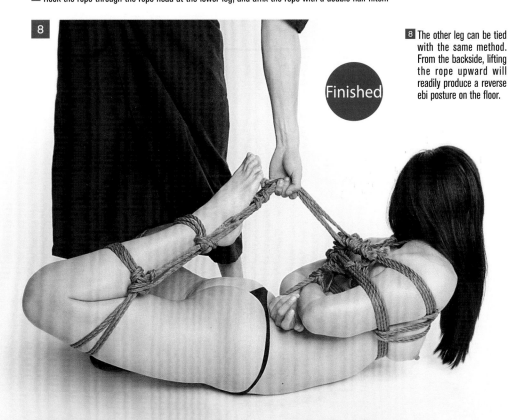

Finished

8 The other leg can be tied with the same method. From the backside, lifting the rope upward will readily produce a reverse ebi posture on the floor.

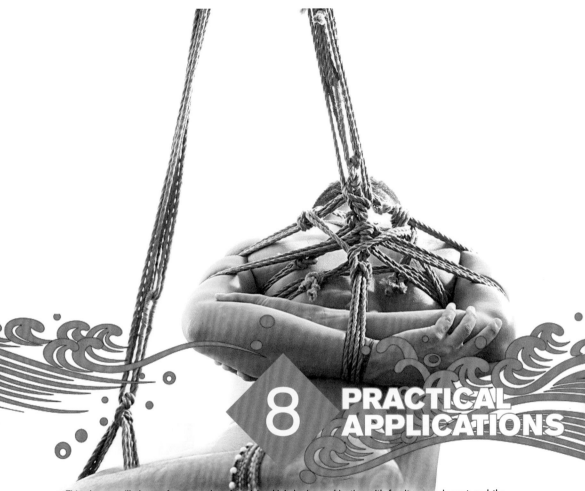

8 PRACTICAL APPLICATIONS

This chapter will show a few examples of applying kinbaku in combination with furniture, equipment, and the location you are playing in. In practice, you may encounter countless situations. The purpose of this book is not to provide bondage routines for you to follow rigidly. Instead, I will use these examples to demonstrate some general principles.

In practical application, kinbaku is bound to have some element of improvisation. The Rope Top may first conceive a general posture, and then start tying from the most obvious starting point. Then they will observe the status of the Rope Bottom, and make adjustments accordingly. When the bondage is proceeding smoothly, things like what to tie next and which parts should be affixed to one another will naturally surface. When you achieve a certain rhythm of bondage, you may feel that this is a successful kinbaku session.

From the beginning, many people are attracted to the unique aesthetics and ambience of Japanese rope bondage. In this book, we have discussed kinbaku done for the sake of delightfulness, classic restraint positions, and how to weave beautiful rope decorations. We have also discussed many safety rules, as well as intimacy and communication during kinbaku. However, for those who are drawn to SM and more intense bondage, we have prepared for you the last section – "Semenawa."

8.1 Application of Furniture

When tying the Rope Bottom to furniture or other fixtures, my principle is: if there are many points on the fixture to attach the rope, choose the points that are closer to the Rope Bottom. Rather than expending the rope to wrap around furniture, it is better to let the rope exert its effect on the Rope Bottom as much as possible. You can use the rope to tie their body directly, hook the ropes they are already tied with to tighten their bondage, or create sensations by laying the rope across them. Devote your attention to the person you are tying instead of the rope or the furniture.

Chair

1 In this example, we start with the right wrist of the Rope Bottom. Tie her right hand by using a method that is similar to the thigh tie (Section 6.4).

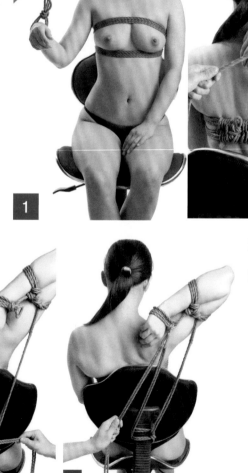

2 Affix the rope to the back of the chair.

3 Rather than tying to the furniture, hook the working end onto the rope on the bottom's hand, to further pull on her body.

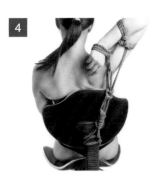

4 Tie off the rope.

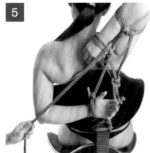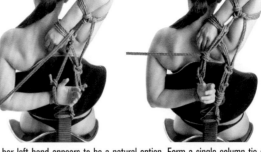

5 Tying her left hand appears to be a natural option. Form a single column tie on her left wrist, hook the working end onto the rope on her right arm, and tie off the rope.

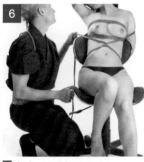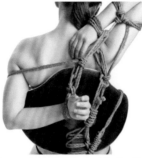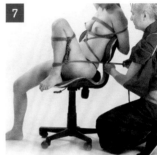

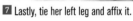

6 Us the remaining rope to wrap around the rope bottom's waist, and finally affix the rope onto the back of the chair.

7 Lastly, tie her left leg and affix it.

Finished

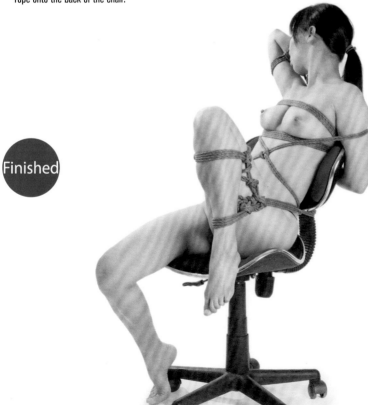

Table

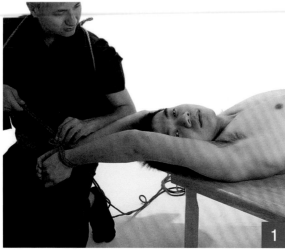 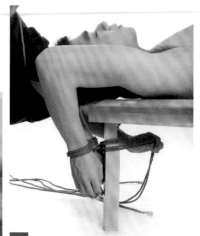

1 Start with a single column tie around both wrists.

2 Fasten the rope to a table leg that is close to you.

3 Since there is still some leftover rope, use it to fasten the rope bottom's upper arms that are close by.

4 The next obvious target for tying is legs. Perhaps this time you may tie each leg separately on the two sides of the table. Start by forming a single column tie around an ankle.

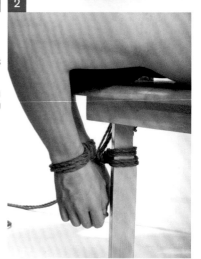

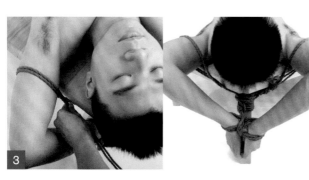 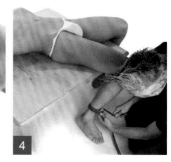

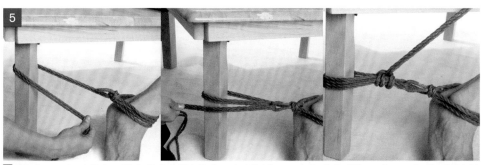

5 Affix the rope to a table leg with double half hitch. To the extent that the rope bottom's flexibility can bear, make him stretch his limbs as much as possible.

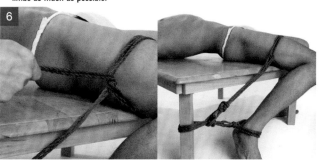

6 Do not waste the leftover rope on the furniture. Let's grab his thigh.

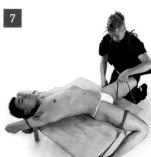

7 Use the same method to tie his other side. Of course, you can also try some asymmetrical posture.

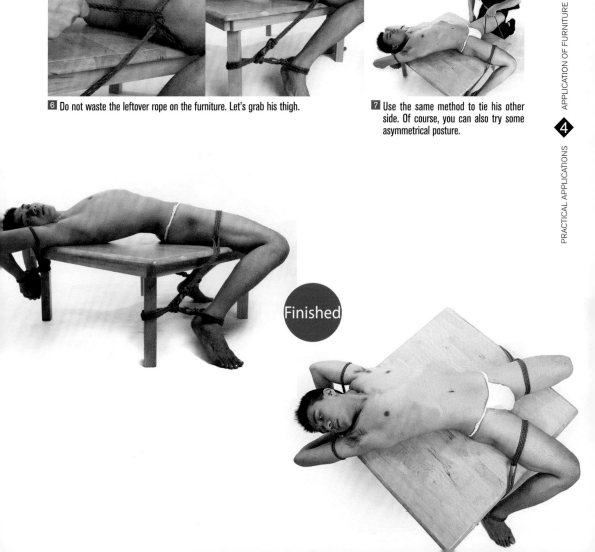

Finished

8.2 Application of Suspension Points

I do not intend to cover full suspension in this book. However, if there is some suspension point to support body weight, you don't have to lift the Rope Bottom off the ground to come up with many variations of bondage. This section will demonstrate a few ways to use suspension points for partial suspension.

In Taiwan, most homes do not have a beam that can be used to hang a suspension ring. When one wants to have a suspension point, if drilling in the ceiling is not an option, then the only way is to use the dungeon equipment in the few adult-themed hotels. Let's emphasize the safety issues that has been mentioned previously. Some indoor equipment may look sturdy, but is in fact merely decoration that cannot bear weight. Door frames and clothes stands also cannot bear a lot of weight. Carabiners must be of specialist quality, the kind whose safety rating has been certified. Ornamental carabiners sold in stationary stores must not be used.

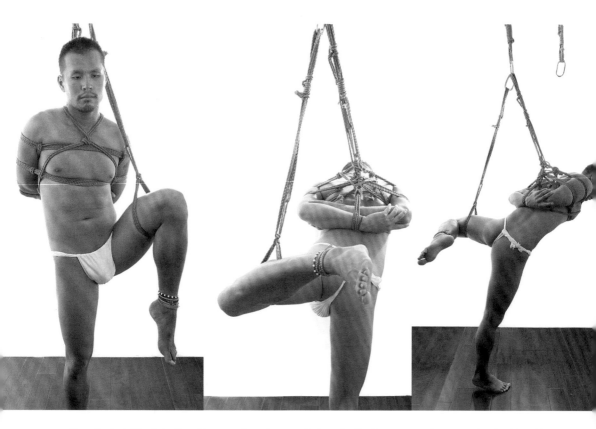

From the backside of the Rope Bottom, pull up the upper body, and affix the rope onto the suspension ring. Then lift one leg. At this time, the Rope Bottom's chest and genitals are defenseless. This is a posture that is very suitable for whipping the butt, or playing with the sensitive parts. During struggle, the Rope Bottom can easily lose balance. At this time, you can encourage the Rope Bottom to give up standing on his own, and place his weight on the rope. Surrender the control of balance to the Rope Top. This is why all partial suspension should be prepared as if it could end up as full suspension.

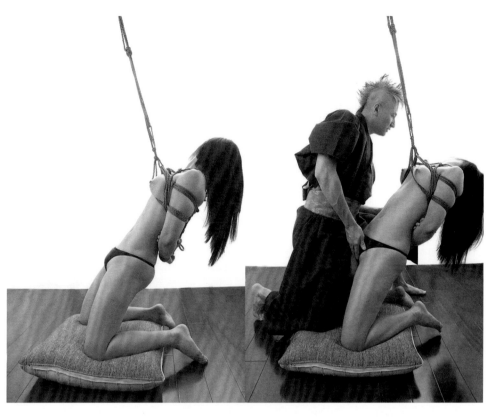

Make the rope bottom kneel on the floor, and pull the body up from the front side. When adopting this posture, you can put a cushion on the floor to make the Rope Bottom's knees more comfortable.

For the postures demonstrated in this section, if a suspension point fails, the rope bottoms cannot protect themselves. Please keep the safety rules in mind, and determine whether the suspension point is firm. You cannot leave the Rope Bottoms by themselves, in case you need to respond to an emergency situation. Prepare equipment such as trauma shears, in order to undo the tie whenever necessary. Be aware that this play can be dangerous, and should only be undertaken if the rope Top has the skill, the suspension point and tools are appropriate, and the Rope Bottom is aware of the risks involved.

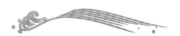

8.3 About Semenawa

From the beginning to the end, this book emphasizes safety and comfort, treating kinbaku as a delightful pursuit, a game, and a way to aid sexual love. The readers may ask: what about SM? Many people are first attracted to SM, and then begin to encounter Japanese kinbaku. After learning many kinbaku techniques, safety issues, and many not-so-hardcore delightful kinbaku skills, we cannot help but asking whether kinbaku has other connotations. What kind of role can rope play in SM?

Indeed, rope bondage is not just a way for restraining; the rope itself can be used as a tool for interrogation, and becomes part of torture. The "ebi-seme" and "suruga-toi" [hands and feet tied behind the victim's back, and hanged from the ceiling with a rock on the back], along with other ties are all rope-based torture techniques of the Edo period. Modern Japanese kinbaku rarely uses the same techniques these days, but nonetheless has derived from these techniques something that embodies Japanese aesthetics.

Even if one follows the safety rules, there are many ways to make the rope bottom suffer. Suspend the rope bottom off the ground, or place his or her weight on the body's sensitive areas. Wrap the rope tightly around a body part, then slap or rub the Rope Bottom's skin. Pull open or compress the Rope Bottom's body, forcing their body into uncomfortable postures. For some postures, the Rope Bottom can only choose between the two agonizing positions. One typical method is to lift up the Rope Bottom so that only the toes are touching the ground. Consequently, standing on toes will make the legs sore, but not using legs to support one's body weight will cause painful pulling by the rope. There are also floor bondage techniques that have similar challenges.

However, semenawa is not just for bringing pain to someone. Abruptly pinching, hitting, or suspending the Rope Bottom is only brutal crudeness, with no aesthetics to speak of. The pursuit of semenawa is a kind of "beauty in suffering."

A seasoned nawashi will first tie up the rope model, and attach the rope to some suspension point or some other fixed object. Then the nawashi will step back and observe them, giving them time to adapt to the rope. Only then will the nawashi add the next piece of rope. The rope model's response will tell the nawashi which part to tie, and where to affix the rope, making sure that each rope, or section of a rope, is being used for a purpose. Perhaps it is to grip him or her tightly, or to suspend them higher, or to stimulate some area.

Layers of adaptation allow for adding new rope, removing a rope, giving them a break, or pushing a rope model to the next boundary. Pulling tight again, or moving into different postures, slowly brings up endorphins. We may see that the rope model is gradually becoming dazed, entering the so-called "rope drunk" state. Only then will the nawashi finally resort to methods such as hot waxing or caning, and make the rope model cry out loud, to bring the semenawa training to its climax. This is "beauty in suffering."

After slowly releasing the rope model and bringing him or her down, it is necessary to comfort, to make peace, and to embrace. Only then will this whole process be brought to its satisfactory conclusion.

Among the Japanese nawashi, people such as Nureki Chimuo, Yukimura Haruki, and Naka Akira are renowned for their interpretations for this style of kinbaku. The Italian rope practitioner Riccardo Wildties is also carrying forward semenawa in Europe.

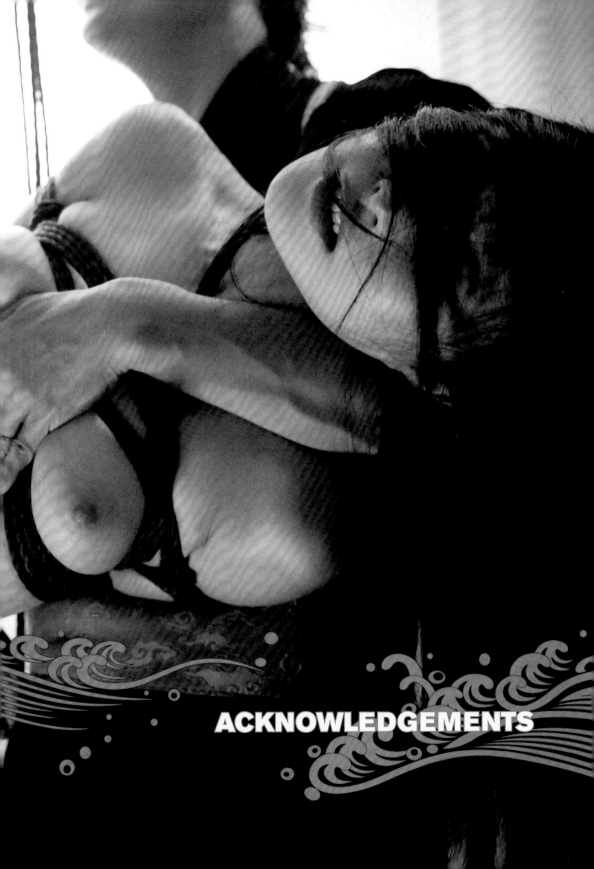

ACKNOWLEDGEMENTS

Acknowledgements

Around mid-2011, with coordination by A-Tsung (Hsia Mu-Tsung), Chu-Tsu from Gbooks (editor-in-chief Shao Chi-Mai) and I started discussing the concept of publishing a book that teaches kinbaku. We originally anticipated finishing an outline around the beginning of the following year. However, I procrastinated for over half a year, and only managed to submit the outline in June of 2012. The first draft of this book was only finished around the beginning of 2013. During my procrastination period, I traveled the world – broadening my outlook, and gaining more experience. Only then did I feel that I had enough preparation to write a solid book on kinbaku. This book contains many pictures, with a complex layout; it is very demanding to edit. Gbooks gave me, as the author, a lot of leeway and respect, and my collaboration with them has been a great pleasure. I am very grateful to Gbooks' Chu-Tsu, Petit, Hsiao Hsiao Hai, and White Rabbit, for their patient waiting, devoted production, and enthusiastic marketing.

My photographer Piez worked hard, and accumulated over 1900 pictures to be sorted through. Yet he methodically handled such an enormous workload in an orderly way, which I greatly admire. I am also grateful to the group of models that helped with the photography project: A-Kung, Tai Tan-Ni, Hsiao Ku, Nancy, and Mi Su, along with the photographers who generously provided their works for the collector's edition of this book: Franco Wang, Chen Yu-Wei, Crystal, Mi Su, and Janric.

Regarding everything I know about kinbaku, it is Kanna who first guided me to enter the world of ropes. Being invited into "Kanna Ichi-mon" (the Kanna school of Kinbaku) was a great honor to a foreigner who doesn't know Japanese. The regular patrons of Succubus brought me a lot of endearing memories. Who can imagine that in an adult bar of a foreign country, one would make so many good friends that would open their hearts to one another? Fujii-san gave me ten pieces of rope to encourage me; this is a very big gift that I still hold and treasure to this day. My practice at Kitagawa Salon was a crucial period when I made a breakthrough in my techniques. Under the guidance of many of my predecessors, I practiced several of my repeatedly-failed techniques until they became mastered – they are now among the fortes of my repertoire. I am grateful to those who have taken good care of us, including Kitagawa, Shioda, and Oni-ku. I am also grateful to Pedro Diniz Reis, my good friend who kept inspiring me during this period of my life.

Since 2011, I have been encouraged by the systematic research and classification of rope bondage in the West, and feel that my horizon has been greatly expanded. The concise advice from Wykd Dave and Clover Brooks has benefited me infinitely. Jack the Whipper, Zahara Froggy, Riccardo Wildties, Redsabbath, Hedwig Ve, and Stefano Laforgia inspired me with their performances on stage, and also provided me with their guidance and suggestions. I am also grateful for their proofreading and review.

I am fortunate to become a member of BDSM Company Taiwan. Entering its tenth year, this organization combined everyone's strengths, and has accomplished many things that were unthinkable in those years. Thank you to every member of BDSM Company Taiwan. I am also thankful for Hsiao Mei, de Zuvia, Sheng Wei, Lina, Fox, Five Five, and others, for their critiques and many suggestions in the drafts of this book, along with Key and Wang Hsiao-Chung for their medical consultation. For things regarding kinbaku, I trust Mai Maya's comments the most. Thanks to her introducing me to Hajime Kinoko, I had the opportunity to perform at Toubaku, along with the various subsequent developments. Thank you Nancy. Regarding this book – from handling administrative affairs to performing as a model – she has always dutifully helped me. She often had a stern look when discussing matters with me, causing others to think that she was a mean girl. With regard to kinbaku, I am grateful that she accompanied me to travel to the ends of world, overcame all kinds of difficulties, and accomplished the goals that only we could accomplish. Everything is worth it in the end.

Thank you Akaneko, for being my companion all the way from Europe to Japan to Taiwan. In Tokyo, we explored Succubus together. You were my interpreter in classes, and my partner in practice. You and I grew together at Kitagawa Salon, and you endured with me my most difficult bottleneck period. You came with me to Taiwan, a foreign land for you. You handled the domestic affairs at our home, and laid my worries to rest. You spent the prime of your life with me. I am very fortunate to be with you.

Shin Nawakiri

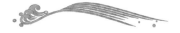

About BDSM Company Taiwan

www.bdsm.com.tw

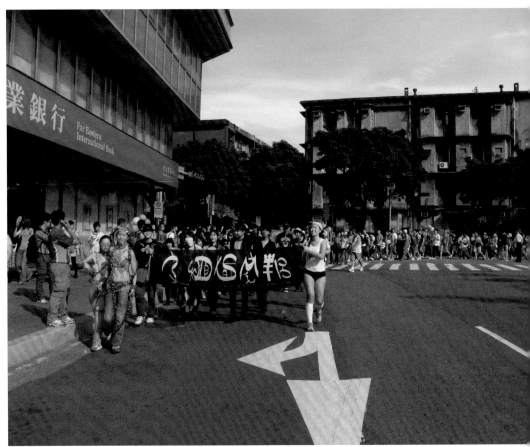

皮繩愉虐邦參加 2009 年同志大遊行。

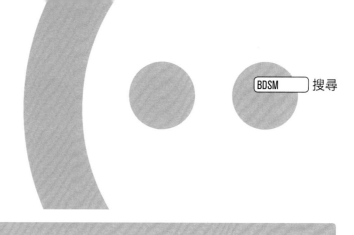

BDSM Company Taiwan is a social movement and performing group. We pay close attention to issues relating to BDSM and gender equality, and are active in multi-sexual artistic performances.

Our members come from every corner of society, with all kinds of professions and trades. Regardless of who each of us are – performing artists, students, office workers, designers – we all have something in common: we all love BDSM, and harbor the ambition to spread the joy of SM to the wider world. Through our various public meetings and activities, we actively seek to unite the SM community in Taiwan. We strive for opportunities for SM enthusiasts to advocate in public and gain the rights to express their sexuality. We also connect with the various groups from the LGBTQ movement, while promoting LGBTQ positions and gender equality in Taiwan.

In addition, we also publish books, take actions, and put on performances, in order to represent BDSM culture to the general public as a form of art. Whether it is teaching bondage skills, or telling the various LGBTQ people's life stories on stage, we hope to bring BDSM into public view. We hope to help everyone personally experience the fact that – in this world – there are many different types of love and different manifestations of desire.

Biographies

Author
Shin Nawakiri

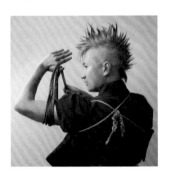

A student of Nawashi Kanna in Tokyo, Shin Nawakiri began his studies of kinbaku in 2003. One of the founders of BDSM Company Taiwan in 2004, this organization was the first support group to publicly advocate for BDSM rights in Taiwan, dedicated to building sexuality communities and strengthening them. From 2006 to 2010, he began participating in the local "Dancing Rope Maiden" performances, before his 2011 debut as an international kinbaku performance artist. Beginning in Tokyo, his artistry has led to him performing and teaching in Macao, Tapei, Moscow, London, and beyond. You can learn more about Shin at http://bittersweet.asia/

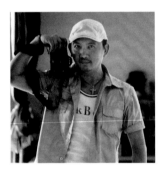

Photographer
Piez Jeng

Piez Jeng began his pursuit of photographing the human form while still in school. An expert at using light and shadow to sculpt the figure, he applies numerous classical and modern techniques to produce engaging images. Despite the popularity of digital photography these days, Piez insists on traditional approaches to create his themed photographic aesthetics. He believes in helping his models present their own multifaceted characters, which distinguishes him from the singular standard of commercial photography. In addition to his work with models, Piez has been involved in design, illustration, creative work, and other photography for over ten years. His website is http://piezphoto.com/

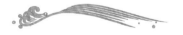